cardiology
cases

cardiology cases

40 Cases

Clinical Discussions for Medical Students and Residents

Emphasis on the Pathophysiology of Disease

JORGE C. RIOS MD, FACC, FACP
GREGORIO KOSS MD, FACC
NANCY SELFRIDGE MD

Copyright © 2018 by Jorge Rios.

Library of Congress Control Number: 2018906577
ISBN: Hardcover 978-1-9845-3119-3
Softcover 978-1-9845-3118-6
eBook 978-1-9845-3117-9

All rights reserved. No part of this book may be reproduced or transmitted in any form or by any means, electronic or mechanical, including photocopying, recording, or by any information storage and retrieval system, without permission in writing from the copyright owner.

Any people depicted in stock imagery provided by Getty Images are models, and such images are being used for illustrative purposes only. Certain stock imagery © Getty Images.

Print information available on the last page.

Rev. date: 07/28/2018

To order additional copies of this book, contact:
Xlibris
1-888-795-4274
www.Xlibris.com
Orders@Xlibris.com

CONTENTS

ACKNOWLEDGMENT xi
INTRODUCTION xiii
CASE NO. 1: FUNCTIONAL MURMUR—
   REVIEW OF BASIC CONCEPTS 1
CASE 1 QUESTIONS... 14

VALVULAR HEART DISEASE

CASE NO. 2: MITRAL STENOSIS 18
CASE 2 QUESTIONS... 26
CASE NO. 3: CHRONIC MITRAL REGURGITATION 28
CASE 3 QUESTIONS... 37
CASE NO. 4: ACUTE MITRAL REGURGITATION 39
CASE 4 QUESTIONS... 43
CASE NO. 5: MITRAL VALVE PROLAPSE 45
CASE 5 QUESTIONS... 48
CASE NO. 6: TRICUSPID REGURGITATION 49
CASE 6 QUESTIONS... 53
CASE NO. 7: VALVULAR AORTIC STENOSIS.................. 54
CASE 7 QUESTIONS... 64
CASE NO. 8: CHRONIC AORTIC REGURGITATION 66

CASE 8 QUESTIONS..74
CASE NO. 9: ACUTE AORTIC REGURGITATION..............76
CASE 9 QUESTIONS..81

CORONARY DISEASE

MYOCARDIAL ISCHEMIA

CASE NO 10: STABLE ANGINA PECTORIS 84
CASE 10 QUESTIONS..95
CASE NO. 11: ACUTE MYOCARDIAL INFARCTION 97
CASE 11 QUESTIONS... 114
CASE NO. 12: VENTRICULAR ANEURYSM..................... 116
CASE 12 QUESTIONS... 119
CASE NO. 13: UNSTABLE ANGINA 121
CASE 13 QUESTIONS... 125
CASE NO. 14: ACUTE MI AND HEART BLOCK............... 127
CASE 14 QUESTIONS... 134
CASE NO. 15: ACUTE MI HYPOTENSION-
    CARDIOGENIC SHOCK.. 136
CASE 15 QUESTIONS... 142
CASE NO. 16: ACUTE MYOCARDIAL
    INFARCTION—
    HYPOTENSION 144
CASE 16 QUESTIONS... 148
CASE NO. 17: UNSTABLE ANGINA PECTORIS 149
CASE 17 QUESTIONS...155

CASE NO. 18: ORTHOSTATIC HYPOTENSION
   IN A POST-MI HYPERTENSIVE PATIENT 157
CASE 18 QUESTIONS 165
CASE NO 19: POST-MI VENTRICULAR TACHYCARDIA 166
CASE 19 QUESTIONS 174

CARDIOMYOPATHIES

HEART FAILURE

CASE NO. 20: POSTPARTUM HEART
   FAILURE—DILATED CARDIOMYOPATHY 178
CASE 20 QUESTIONS 184
CASE NO. 21: HYPERTENSION—DIASTOLIC
   HEART FAILURE 186
CASE 21 QUESTIONS 196
CASE NO. 22: RESTRICTIVE CARDIOMYOPATHY 197
CASE 22 QUESTIONS 201
CASE NO. 23: OBSTRUCTIVE CARDIOMYOPATHY 202
CASE 23 QUESTIONS 207

PERICARDIAL DISEASE

CASE NO. 24: CARDIAC TAMPONADE 210
CASE 24 QUESTIONS 216
CASE NO. 25. CONSTRICTIVE PERICARDITIS 218
CASE 25 QUESTIONS 222

CARDIAC ARRHYTHMIAS

CASE NO. 26: COMPLETE HEART BLOCK	226
CASE 26 QUESTIONS	236
CASE NO. 27: BRADYARRHYTHMIAS—SICK SINUS SYNDROME	237
CASE 27 QUESTIONS	240
CASE NO. 28: WENCKEBACH PHENOMENA	241
CASE 28 QUESTIONS	245
CASE NO. 29: MOBITZ 2	246
CASE 29 QUESTIONS	250
CASE NO. 30: SUPRAVENTRICULAR TACHYCARDIA	252
CASE 30 QUESTIONS	257
CASE NO. 31: WOLFF-PARKINSON-WHITE SYNDROME	259
CASE 31 QUESTIONS	263
CASE NO. 32: ATRIAL FIBRILLATION	264
CASE 32 QUESTIONS	271
CASE NO. 33: ATRIAL FLUTTER	272
CASES 32–33 QUESTIONS	276
CASE NO. 34: LONG QT INTERVAL	278
CASE 34 QUESTIONS	283

CONGENITAL HEART DISEASE

CASE NO. 35: PATHOPHYSIOLOGY OF LEFT TO RIGHT SHUNTS—VENTRICULAR SEPTAL DEFECT	286
CASE 35 QUESTIONS	292

CASE NO. 36: ATRIAL SEPTAL DEFECT..........................293
CASE 36 QUESTIONS..297
CASE NO. 37: PATENT DUCTUS ARTERIOSUS.............298
CASE 37 QUESTIONS..302
CASE NO. 38: CONGENITAL CARDIAC
    DEFECT AND PULMONARY HYPERTENSION 304
CASE 38 QUESTIONS..310
CASE NO. 39: CYANOTIC HEART DISEASE—
    TETRALOGY OF FALLOT 312
CASE 39 QUESTIONS..317
CASE NO. 40: PULMONARY STENOSIS 318
CASE 40 QUESTIONS..322
CORRECT ANSWERS...323
SELECTED REFERENCES..325
INDEX..365

ACKNOWLEDGMENT

To the many patients that over many years allowed our students to learn by hearing their medical secrets and their physical finding continued to give us the inspirations.

To the thousands of students that over the many years continued to give us the inspiration to do what we did

To our families, that always provided us the support to continue doing what we have loved the most

INTRODUCTION

Medical education has changed. The artificial division between basic sciences and clinical sciences practiced in medical schools has eroded and is replaced by teaching approaches where clinical examples are used to explain the application of basic science principles and vice versa. At the same time, clinical discussions often include reviews of the basic sciences taught earlier during the first years of medical school. This approach facilitates understanding of the mechanism of diseases and provides a more scientific content.

We hope to achieve the same goal, presenting actual clinical cases that allow *review of* basic concepts and principles of cardiac physiology and how they explain the pathophysiology applicable to the case.

This is not a textbook. We will present cardiac cases that represent various pathologies encountered in clinical practice. These cases are often encountered in the daily clinical setting or discussed on bedside rounds or in resident reports. Our emphasis is on the mechanism of disease and alterations on physiology with minimal discussion on the diagnostic technology commonly used. The content of each case will prepare the resident or student for the discussion likely to happen in those settings.

At the end of each case, we will present a number of practice questions relevant to the manifestations of the disease and the pathophysiology. Answers will be found in a separate chapter at the end.

We have included references. We present a list of traditional textbooks that can provide greater depth in the discussion, and for each case, we offer a list of articles that allow more extensive review of each topic.

We hope that students and residents find this book useful and practical.

CASE NO. 1: FUNCTIONAL MURMUR—REVIEW OF BASIC CONCEPTS

A twenty-five-year-old female on the third trimester of an uncomplicated pregnancy is seen by her obstetrician. Her past medical history is noncontributory, and on close questioning, she denies any symptoms commonly associated with heart disease. In the past, she had been told by her primary care physician that she had no cardiac murmurs.

On physical examination, heart rate was 100x', no evidence of ventricular hypertrophy, and all pulses were normal but slightly bounding. Jugular pulse was normal. Auscultation revealed a slightly louder S1, normal splitting of S2, and a very soft, low frequency S3. A grade 2 ejection systolic murmur was best heard at the second left interspace without radiation. The remainder of the cardiovascular examination was unremarkable.

ECG and chest x-ray were normal.

DISCUSSION

The clinical presentation and physical findings and her past medical history suggest a normal individual with physiological changes and physical findings associated with pregnancy. We will also review some basic concepts of cardiac physiology learned in the first year of medical school that apply to this and the other cases. They are critical in understanding most cardiac diseases.

What changes in cardiovascular physiology occur during pregnancy?

Pregnancy results in multiple changes in cardiovascular physiology, and they begin as early as the eighth week of pregnancy.

- Cardiac output increases by 20% and up to 40%. The maximum cardiac output is found at about 20–28 weeks' gestation. There is a minimal fall at term.
- The increase in cardiac output results from increased stroke volume and heart rate.
- Peripheral vasodilatation is the most likely cause of changes in cardiac output. Peripheral vascular resistance decreases by 25–30% with the consequent increase in cardiac output.
- These changes are mediated by endothelium-dependent factors, such as nitric oxide synthesis, upregulated by estradiol and possibly prostaglandins.
- Increase in stroke volume is possible due to the early increase in ventricular end-diastolic volume seen in pregnancy.
- The heart is physiologically dilated, and myocardial contractility is increased.
- Although stroke volume declines toward term, the increase in maternal heart rate (10–20 beats per minute) is maintained, thus preserving the increased cardiac output.
- Blood pressure decreases in the first and second trimesters but increases to nonpregnant levels in the third trimester.
- Pulmonary capillary wedge pressure and central venous pressure do not increase significantly.
- Pulmonary vascular resistance (PVR), like systemic vascular resistance (SVR), decreases significantly.

- Serum osmotic pressure is reduced by 10–15%.
- Maternal position alters hemodynamics in advanced pregnancy. In the supine position, pressure of the uterus on the inferior vena cava (IVC) causes a reduction in venous return to the heart and a potential fall in cardiac output.
- After delivery, cardiac output increases, followed by a rapid decline to prepartum values.

The above physiological changes affect findings in the cardiovascular examination that may be misinterpreted as pathological, such as

- Bounding or collapsing arterial pulse.
- An ejection systolic murmur, present in over 90% of pregnant women. The murmur may be loud and audible all over the precordium.
- A loud first heart sound caused by increased contractility.
- A third heart sound secondary to increased cardiac output.
- A continuous murmur over breast tissue secondary to increased flow over the breasts.

The discussion above motivates a review of some basic physiological concepts applicable to day-to-day clinical practice.

CARDIAC OUTPUT

Cardiac output is expressed in liters per minute and is calculated through various methods (Fick principle, thermodilution, echocardiography, etc.).

The main factors that determine cardiac output include heart rate and stroke volume.

REGULATION OF THE HEART RATE

The regulation of heart rate rests on parasympathetic and sympathetic effects.

- At rest, balance between parasympathetic and sympathetic maintains heart rate down to around 60–70 beats per minute. At night, further decrease in heart rate can be noted.
- An increase in heart rate is secondary to the release of norepinephrine that increases the slope of phase 4 of the pacemaker potential by opening Ca^{++} channels. The pacemaker reaches threshold potential faster, and the heart rate is increased.

REGULATION OF STROKE VOLUME

Stroke volume is the amount of blood discharged by the ventricle on each systole and is calculated. as

Stroke volume = cardiac output / heart rate

What are important factors that influence stroke volume?

- *Sympathetic effect.* Norepinephrine increases the force of contraction by increasing the Ca^{++} effect. This would increase ejection fraction and stroke volume.
- *Afterload.* Aortic pressure is referred as **afterload** because it is the load experienced by the ventricle after it begins contracting.
- *Frank-Starling mechanism.* Heart muscle fibers respond to stretch by increasing contractility. Changes in the end-diastolic volume result in an increase in stroke volume due to an increased expenditure of ATP.

What other factors influence contractility? How is contractility changed?

The release of catecholamine determines the concentration of calcium ions in a cardiac muscle cell. The increased force of contraction depends on the concentration of calcium ions in the cell. This results in increased binding of myosin and actin.

Some factors in the control of contractility include the following:

- *Increased circulating levels of catecholamines.* This causes the receptors to activate adenylate cyclase and increase CAM, phosphorylating phospholamban (via protein kinase A).
- *Phosphorylating phospholamban.* When phospholamban is not phosphorylated, it inhibits the calcium pumps. When levels of calcium stored in the sarcoplasmic reticulum are increased, it allows a higher rate of calcium release at the next contraction.
- Troponin-C is sensitized to the effects of calcium.
- Phosphorylating L-type calcium channels increase the permeability to calcium, increasing contractility.

Changes in cardiac contractility shift the entire Frank-Starling curve. The curve shifts upward when contractility increases and downward if contractility decreases.

How are changes in contractility influence clinical examination?

- Increased contractility results in faster upstroke of the ventricular pressure curve during isometric contraction. This is often accompanied by a brisk, faster arterial pulse upstroke.

- S1 is louder. The loudest component of S1 is related to closure of the mitral and tricuspid valves. Softer, lower frequency components are caused by myocardial contractility. In the case of increase rate of contractility, such as exercise or anemia, the myocardial component of the first sound increases in intensity.

Why is there a difference in timing in the closure of aortic and pulmonary valves?

The left ventricular wall faces a stronger resistance and creates stronger contractile force than that of the right ventricle, resulting in earlier closure. Also, the inspiratory changes in right ventricular volume change during causes an increased duration of systole.

ADDITIONAL SOUNDS GENERATED

A supple ventricular myocardium undergoes rapid expansion, creating a low frequency sound at the end of rapid ventricular filling. An S3 is a normal finding in young people, especially those with a high cardiac output state. S4 is not observed in normal individuals since it represents decreased compliance of the ventricles.

THE PRESSURE VOLUME CURVE

The pressure/volume curve is a simple and graphic way to describe the changes in pressure and volume occurring during the cardiac cycle.

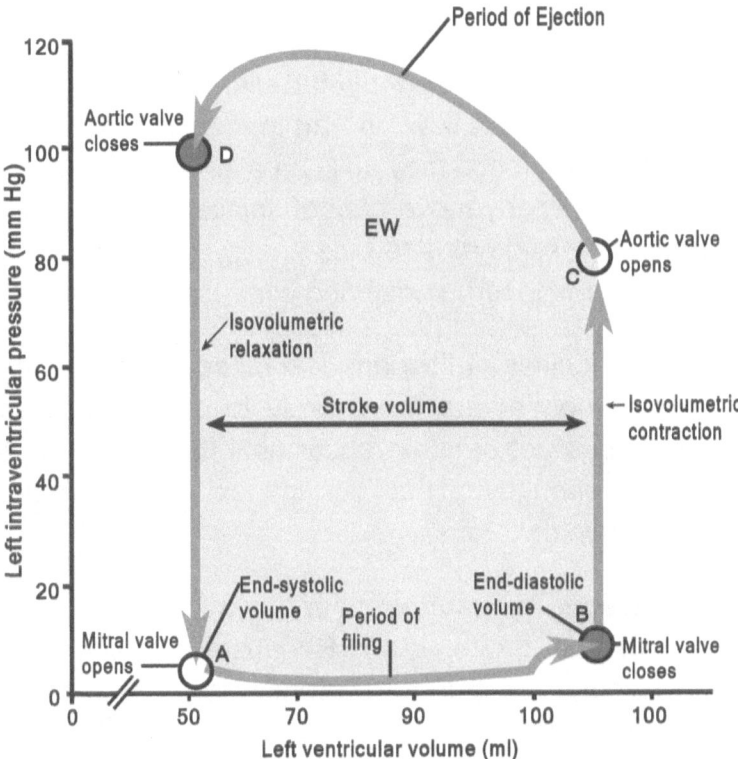

Fig. 1.1. In the horizontal axis, we observe changes in ventricular volume and changes in pressure in the vertical axis. The stroke volume is represented by the volume changes between isovolumetric contraction and isovolumetric relaxation.

Understanding the pressure/volume loop facilitates the understanding of the pathophysiology of cardiac lesions. If students understand and remember the pressure/volume curve, they can explain the pathophysiology of most lesions.

How do cardiac murmurs originate?

An early and brief ejection murmur, as observed in pregnancy, is usually not indicative of heart disease, but it is related to increase cardiac flow. The increased flow generates turbulence.

Murmurs are caused by turbulence. Under normal circumstances, blood flow is laminar, characterized by concentric layers of blood moving in parallel down the length of the vessel. The orderly movement of adjacent layers of blood flow through a vessel helps reduce energy loss. Disruption of laminar flow leads to turbulence and increased energy losses.

High velocities of flow and low blood viscosity (occurs with chronic anemia) are more likely to cause turbulence. Turbulence does not begin to occur until the velocity of flow becomes high enough that the flow lamina breaks apart. At this point, turbulence develops.

Turbulence generates sound waves (i.e., ejection murmurs, carotid bruits, etc.). Because higher velocities enhance turbulence, murmurs intensify as flow increases. These can result from

- high cardiac output, even across anatomically normal valves;
- a decrease in blood viscosity; and
- increasing degree of obstruction.

As illustrated by this case, a high cardiac output may cause new and functional murmurs. The increased flow and the decreased viscosity are proper explanations of the origin of the murmur.

When does the highest flow velocity occur in a healthy heart?

Velocity of flow is at its highest in the first half of systole. That explains the development of turbulence and the development of a functional murmur in early systole.

Several other hemodynamic calculations are commonly used and are of special significance in understanding the pathophysiology of cardiac diseases. The student will encounter application of these concepts especially while rotating through intensive care or cardiac care units.

- **Cardiac output** is the amount of blood the heart pumps in one minute, expressed in liters per minute.

Related calculations derived from cardiac output determinations include the following:

- **Cardiac index** expresses cardiac output as a function of body surface area. The formula is as follows:

Cardiac output (liters/minute) / body surface area (in m2)

- **Stroke volume** is the amount ejected from the ventricles per heartbeat. The formula is as follows:

Cardiac output (liter per minute) / heart rate (beats per minute)

If the calculation is based on echocardiography, the formula is as follows:

Stroke volume = end diastolic volume - end systolic volume

Stroke index is the stroke volume corrected for body surface area. *Formula is as follows:*

Stroke volume / body surface area (in m2)

Ejection fraction is the percentage of ventricular volume ejected during each systole. The formula is as follows:

Ejection fraction = stroke volume (cc per beat) / end diastolic volume (cc) × 100, expressed as percentage of end-diastolic volume

Compliance is the property of a material of undergoing elastic deformation and is equal to the reciprocal of stiffness.

Compliance is an important concept in human physiology, and it applies to the ventricles, the atria, as well as the pericardium, lungs, the pleura—all affected by changes in pressure and volume.

Using the left ventricle as an example, if the chamber dilates but diastolic pressure remains low, that means that the ventricle has increased its compliance (i.e., mitral regurgitation). The opposite is if the ventricular volume does not change much but its diastolic pressure increases, that is decreased compliance.

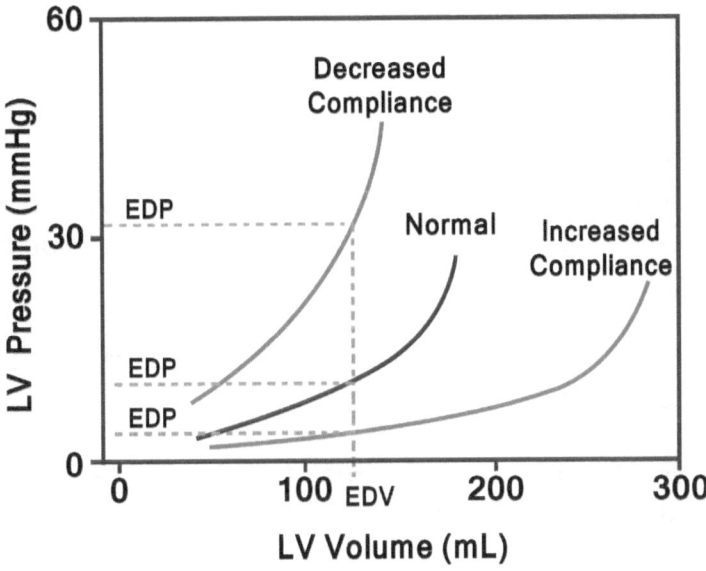

Fig. 1.2. Pressure (y-axis) versus volume (x-axis) illustrates compliance.

Peripheral vascular resistance (PVR) or *total peripheral resistance* (TPR) is the resistance offered to blood flow by the systemic vasculature.

The major regulator of vascular resistance is the vessel radius. Resistance is inversely proportional to the fourth power of the radius of vessels; therefore, small changes in diameter result in large increases or decreases in vascular resistance.

Regulation of vessel radius is a major factor in determining resistance. There is very little pressure change as blood flows from the aorta to the large arteries, but the small arteries and arterioles are the main regulators of TPR.

Vasoconstriction increases TPR, and vasodilation decreases TPR. Exercise and neuronal and hormonal signals, including binding of norepinephrine and epinephrine to the α1 receptor on vascular smooth muscles, cause either vasoconstriction or vasodilation.

The formula is as follows:

Total peripheral resistance = mean systolic blood pressure - central venous pressure (mm Hg) / cardiac output (l per min)

Vascular resistance is a good estimator of afterload (to be discussed later)

Pulmonary vascular resistance is the resistance to flow in the pulmonary system. The formula is as follows:

Mean pulmonary artery pressure (mm Hg) - mean left atrial pressure (or capillary wedge pressure) / cardiac output (l per min)

In a normal circulation, pulmonary vascular resistance is about 20% of systemic resistance. Pulmonary arterioles undergo vasoconstriction as a result of hypoxia, resulting in reduced blood flow. This is the primary process that actively regulates the blood flow distribution in pulmonary tissue. Pulmonary vasculature is also modulated by a variety of other physiological stimuli, but hypoxic vasoconstriction represents the most important process.

Afterload is the load against which the heart contracts to eject blood.

In the systemic circulation, afterload is the pressure that the left ventricular muscle must overcome to eject blood. Elevating arterial systolic pressure or obstructing ventricular ejection increases afterload. Vasodilatation of the arterial tree decreases afterload.

Preload is defined as the end diastolic volume that stretches the right or left ventricle to its greatest dimensions. For example, low venous return lowers right ventricular volume and decreases preload of the right ventricle. In turn, low right ventricular volume deceases left ventricular preload.

Preload is also affected by the following:

- *Respiration.* Intrathoracic pressure decreases during inspiration, and abdominal pressure increases, squeezing local abdominal veins, allowing thoracic veins to expand and increase blood flow toward the right atrium.
- *Skeletal muscles.* The deep vein surrounded by leg muscles squeezes veins and pumps blood back toward the heart.

As we discuss individual cases, we will be referring to these concepts and definitions since they are fundamental to understand the various cardiovascular diseases and their pathophysiology. We encourage that you understand and remember these concepts since it will greatly facilitate knowing and remembering the mechanism of cardiac diseases.

CASE 1 QUESTIONS

1. The rate of ejection (volume/time) in a normal individual occurs is highest in

    a. Uniformly throughout systole
    b. Mid systole
    c. Late systole
    d. Early systole

2. The mechanism of the ejection murmur in this patient is

    a. Valvular incompetence
    b. Valvular calcification
    c. Laminar flow
    d. Turbulent flow

3. The intensity of the ejection murmur will increase with

    a. Hypovolemia
    b. Increased blood velocity
    c. Resting
    d. Fluid overload

4. Functional ejection murmurs

    a. Have fixed intensity
    b. Are not affected by preload
    c. Are not affected by afterload
    d. Will begin when turbulent flow develops

5. In a normal subject, the increased intensity of S1 results from

    a. Undiagnosed aortic stenosis
    b. Increased contractility

c. Abnormal mitral valve opening
d. Abnormal tricuspid valve

6. In this patient, an S3 is caused by

   a. Decreased ventricular compliance
   b. Increased ventricular compliance
   c. Rapid ventricular filling and normal myocardium
   d. Tricuspid regurgitation

7. Administration of a drug that dilates the peripheral vascular tree will

   a. Not affect left heart pressure
   b. Increase systemic resistance
   c. Decrease systemic resistance
   d. Not affect pulmonary resistance

VALVULAR HEART DISEASE

CASE NO. 2: MITRAL STENOSIS

Mrs. ED presented with the classical manifestations of rheumatic mitral stenosis. A forty-eight-year-old female with a history of rheumatic heart disease, she was diagnosed approximately ten years before as having mild mitral stenosis. All these years, she had been active, employed full-time, and capable of carrying all normal activities of daily life.

In the last year, she had noted that her exercise capacity was somewhat limited after moderate physical exercise—for example, she was not capable of running up three flights of steps and had to do it slowly and would stop midway to rest.

Late one night, after sexual activity, she became acutely short of breath, coughing and producing pinkish nonproductive expectoration. Few minutes before, she had noted a very rapid and irregular heartbeat.

She was transported to an emergency department, where the following findings were reported:

- Heart rate at 150 beats per minute—irregular
- Lungs—bilateral basilar rales and diffuse wheezes
- Cardiac examination are as follows:
    - A small apical pulse.
    - Palpable right ventricular lift.
    - Auscultation demonstrates a prominent S1, loud P2, and a diastolic low frequency rumble without presystolic accentuation.

Mitral stenosis results in some classical changes in the chest x-ray as shown below, demonstrating left atrial enlargement, pulmonary congestion, pulmonary edema, and right ventricular hypertrophy.

An ECG (obtained later) shows normal sinus rhythm, left atrial enlargement, and right ventricular hypertrophy—common findings in patients with mitral stenosis.

In patients with mitral stenosis, the echocardiogram commonly demonstrates a narrow and often calcified mitral valve, increased left atrial size, and depending on the pulmonary hypertension, right ventricular hypertrophy.

DISCUSSION

Mitral stenosis is almost always caused by rheumatic fever occurring in years past. Rheumatic fever has decreased dramatically in the US and remains a subtropical disease affecting lower socioeconomic groups. Recent estimates suggest that 15.6 million people worldwide have rheumatic heart disease and that 470,000 new cases of rheumatic fever (approximately 60% of whom will develop rheumatic heart disease) occur annually.

Acute rheumatic fever (ARF) is an autoimmune inflammatory process that develops as a sequela of a streptococcal infection. Patients that acquire rheumatic fever have an abnormal immune response and both B- and T-cells that are unable to distinguish between the invading microbe and certain host tissues.

From the episode of rheumatic fever to the clinical symptoms of mitral stenosis, one or two decades will pass. The initial inflammation will lead to fusion of the leaflets of causing an obstruction of forward flow from left atria to left ventricle.

What are the pathophysiological consequences of mitral stenosis?

In the case being discussed, the acute onset shortness of breath and history of gradual decrease in exercise capacity can be easily explained by the pathophysiology resulting from a stenotic mitral valve.

Once the narrowing of the mitral valve proceeds from a normal opening of 4–6 to a narrow orifice of 2 cm^2, a pressure gradient between left atria and left ventricle will develop, as shown in the enclosed figure.

The impairment in forward flow across the obstructed mitral valve results in elevation of left atrial pressure. As the heart rate increases, the diastolic filling period is shorter, and this will lead to greater elevation in atrial pressure.

What happens then?

The elevated capillary pressure will increase hydrostatic pressure in the pulmonary capillary, allowing fluid to transudate across the alveoli membrane and collect in the lungs, explaining the pulmonary edema.

The alveoli filled with fluid will cause abnormalities in gas exchange, affecting diffusion of O_2. Cyanosis is a common observation in mitral stenosis resulting from the * abnormal O_2 diffusion (central cyanosis).

The dyspnea results from the elevation of left atrial pressure, causing alveolar transudates that impairs ventilation and perfusion.

The decrease in cardiac output is easily explained by examining the pressure volume loop.

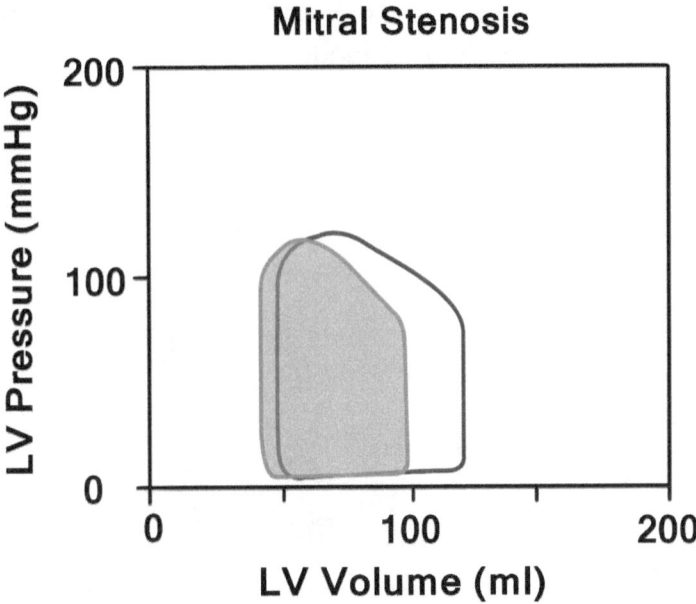

Fig. 2.3. Pressure/volume curve in a patient with mitral stenosis showing lowered preload, decreased left ventricular filling, decreased stroke volume, lower LV systolic pressure, and decreased end-diastolic left ventricular volume.

The physiological changes explain the physical findings seen in patients with mitral stenosis.

- *Loud S1.* The elevation of atrial pressure will delay the closing of the mitral valve, and it will occur at a time that when the rate of the ventricular contraction has increased the velocity of closure of the mitral valve. **As a result, the intensity of S1 will increase**—a classical finding in mitral stenosis

- *Opening snap.* The opening of the mitral valve and tension on the fused leaflets cause the opening snap. The mitral valve will open when ventricular pressure falls below atrial pressure. As you can conclude from observing the illustration, the higher the left atrial pressure, the earlier the opening snap in closer proximity of the second heart sound.

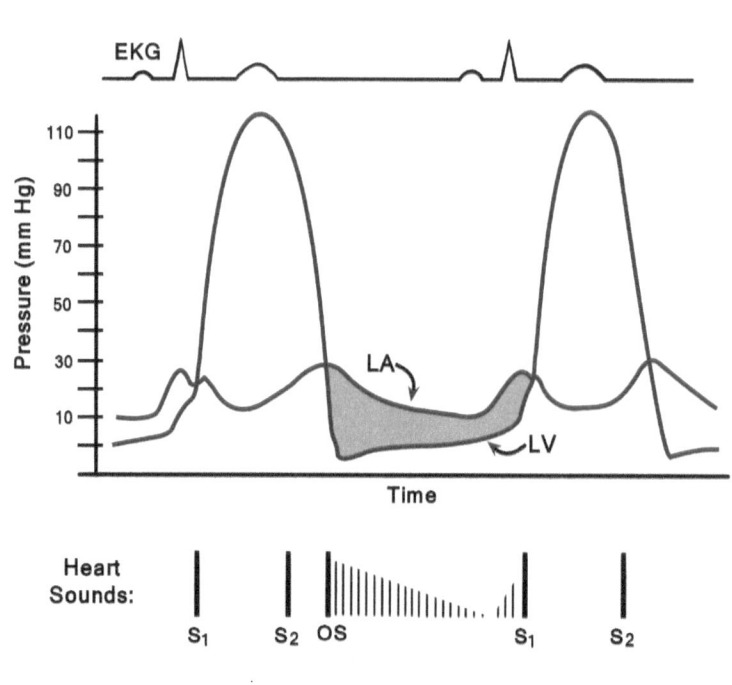

Fig. 2.7. Tracing of left atrial and left ventricular pressure. Shaded in diastole is the pressure gradient across the mitral valve as a result of the stenosis. Note that at end of diastole, synchronous to the P wave of the ECG, the gradient increases and would result in an accentuation of the murmur.

- *Atrial pressure and "x" descent.* The "x" descent of the left atrial pressure (the downward slope of the atrial pressure from the peak of the "v" wave) will be slower than normal as a reflection of the difficulty of blood flowing in the left ventricle.
- *Diastolic rumble.* The behavior of the diastolic murmur correlates with the pressure gradient. The intensity will decrease as the pressure in the left atrium descends

and at the end of diastole. In the presence of normal sinus rhythm, atrial contraction will cause an increase in the pressure gradient and intensify the murmur (commonly known as presystolic accentuation). If atrial fibrillation develops, losing atrial contraction makes the presystolic accentuation disappear.

The intensity of the rumble is also influenced by the cardiac output. In severe cases, the gradient may be large and the output (diastolic flow) low, and the murmur may be of very low intensity.

Echocardiography will give good assessments of the mitral valve area, magnitude of the gradient, presence of calcification and atrial thrombi, and estimate level of pulmonary pressure.

The major complicatios of mitral stenosis include the following:

- *Pulmonary hypertension.* This develops as a result of the retrograde transmission of left atrial pressure that causes pulmonary arteriolar vasoconstriction. Initially this pulmonary hypertension will be vaso-reactive and will regress with reduction of atrial pressure.

  Over time, the vaso-reactive hypertension will lead to obliterative changes in the pulmonary vascular bed with hyperplasia of the intima and hypertrophy of the medial muscular layer. The increasing degree of obstruction gradually elevates pulmonary pressure.

  The precise mechanism of pulmonary arterial hypertension is not yet clear, but it is believed that the endothelial dysfunction, caused by the elevated pressure, results in the stimulation of the synthesis of vasoconstrictors such as thromboxane and vascular endothelial growth factor (VEGF).

- *Right ventricular hypertrophy and tricuspid regurgitation.* As pulmonary arterial pressure increases, right ventricular dilation and tricuspid regurgitation may develop, leading to elevated jugular venous pressure, liver congestion, ascites, and pedal edema. The presence of pulmonary hypertension will have a negative effect on prognosis.

- *Atrial fibrillation.* Atrial fibrillation is one of the most serious complications of mitral stenosis and will occur in approximately half of the patients. Atrial fibrillation, if untreated, will cause a very rapid and irregular ventricular rate only controlled by the refractory period of the AV node.

  The rapid ventricular rate decreases diastolic filling time per minute (up to 37%), and there is less time for the emptying of the atria. A shortened diastolic filling period will further elevate LA and capillary pressure and could cause pulmonary edema.

  The incidence of atrial fibrillation in patients with mitral stenosis is 43.6% and is

    ○ higher in females (72.72%) than males (27.27%) and

    ○ higher if mitral valve area < 1 cm^2 (70.4%) as compared to 29.6% in cases of mitral stenosis with mitral valve area > 1 cm^2.

- *Embolizations.* Atrial fibrillation raises the possibility of clots forming, mainly in the left atrial appendage, causing peipheral embolizations.

Systemic embolization will be cerebral (66.66%) or peripheral (33.33%).

- *Endocarditis.* In 2007, the American Heart Association simplified its recommendations. Antibiotics before dental procedures are only recommended for patients with the highest risk of endocarditis, such as those who have a prosthetic heart valve, those who have had a heart valve repaired with prosthetic material, and those with history of endocarditis.

TREATMENT

Treatment of mitral stenosis is surgical, needing either repair or replacement of the valve. Balloon angioplasty is also used in relief of the stenosis.

In the 2014 American Heart Association / American College of Cardiology (AHA/ACC) guidelines, percutaneous mitral balloon valvotomy (PMBV) is recommended if the valve morphology is favorable and the patient does not have left atrial thrombus or moderate to severe (3+ to 4+) mitral regurgitation.

Mitral repair and commissurotomy are preferred treatments, and sometimes replacement of the valve is needed.

CASE 2 QUESTIONS

1. In a patient with mitral stenosis, atrial fibrillation with a ventricular rate that increases from 60x' to 150 x' will

    a. Decrease mean left atrial pressure
    b. Increase mean left ventricular pressure
    c. Will not affect left atrial pressure
    d. Affect length of diastolic time

2. In a patient with mitral stenosis and atrial fibrillation

    a. Left atrial "c" wave is increased
    b. Atrial "a" wave is absent
    c. "x" descent is slower than normal
    d. "x" descent is faster than normal

3. In a patient with mitral stenosis and atrial fibrillation

    a. Diastolic filling period is constant
    b. Systolic period is shorter than diastolic period
    c. AV node refractory period play a role in diastolic filling period
    d. Ventricular rate is not affected by AV node refractory period

4. In a patient with mitral stenosis, acute reduction of afterload

    a. Will improve symptoms
    b. Can induce severe hypotension
    c. Is the treatment of choice
    d. Increase in preload is essential

5. In a patient with mitral stenosis

    a. Hydrostatic pressure in the pulmonary capillaries will increase
    b. Plasma oncotic pressure will increase
    c. Lowering left atrial pressure will increase hydrostatic pressure in the pulmonary capillaries
    d. Oncotic pressure will decrease

6. In a patient in pulmonary edema

    a. Arterial pO_2 is decreased
    b. Arterial pCO_2 often is increased
    c. Arterial pO_2 is often increased
    d. O_2 saturation is increased

CASE NO. 3: CHRONIC MITRAL REGURGITATION

Mr. PB, a fifty-six-year-old attorney, is referred to a cardiologist for evaluation of a cardiac murmur.

He reported that at age eight, he had acute rheumatic fever, and as a result, he developed a heart murmur that was diagnosed as mitral regurgitation. He recovered uneventfully and lived a normal and productive life with no major health issues. A good golfer, he has played for the last forty years, walking the course without difficulties. He also continued to be an avid swimmer, doing two miles on regular basis.

For the last twelve months, he started to notice some decrease in exercise tolerance, having some shortness of breath following a brisk walk of about half a mile.

Past medical history is unremarkable except for the rheumatic fever mentioned

Physical examination is unremarkable except for cardiovascular system that reveals the following:

- Normal jugular venous pulses.
- Apical impulse slightly displaced toward the left axilla.
- Auscultation demonstrated a soft S1, a normal S2, a soft S3, and a gr3/6 pansystolic murmur of high frequency radiating from the apex to the axilla.
- All peripheral pulses were normal.
- No peripheral edema was present.

Diagnostic tests were performed, and the patient was advised to return for regular follow-up. Cardiac surgery and risks and benefits were explained to the patient.

In chronic mitral regurgitation, depending on the magnitude and duration of the regurgitation, the ECG will show left ventricular hypertrophy, and the echocardiogram may show dilated left atria and ventricle, and regurgitation through an abnormal anterior leaflet is also seen.

DISCUSSION

Mitral valve regurgitation is one of the two most common valvular heart diseases and is quite common in the elderly. The prevalence is 2% of the population, affecting males and females equally.

This patient, who came to us late in the progress of the disease, necessitated that surgery be considered and discussed. He represents one of the common presentations of a person with mitral regurgitation of rheumatic origin. A latent period of many years eventually may lead to left ventricular dysfunction.

A brief review of the anatomy will clarify the pathophysiology:

- The mitral valve is attached to the wall between the left atria and ventricle by a fibrous ring.
- The valve has two leaflets, anterior and posterior. The anterior is the largest (about $2/3$ of the circumference of the ring) and a smaller posterior leaflet.
- The anterior leaflet is the most often affected.
- Each leaflet has fibrous strings, the chorda tendineae that attach to the papillary muscles—one attaches to the anterior muscle and the other one to the posterior.

The valvular ring, leaflets, chordae, and papillary muscle constitute the mitral valve apparatus.

The function of the mitral valve (and the tricuspid valve on the right) is to prevent regurgitation from the ventricle to atria during ventricular systole. When the ventricles contract, the tensing of the papillary muscles will maintain the leaflets in position, keeping the orifice closed. If any of the components of the mitral valve apparatus is dysfunctional, the leaflets would fail to properly close the orifice and create regurgitation.

What can produce mitral regurgitation? The causes are multiple and listed in table 3.1.

CAUSES OF MITRAL REGURGITATION

Leaflet	Papillary Muscle
o Rheumatic Fever	o Dysfunction (ischemia/infarct, aneurysm, dilated cardiomyopathy)
o Collage diseases (SLE, scleroderma)	o Rupture (infarction, trauma)
o Connective tissue diseases (Marfan, mitral Valve prolapse)	
o Endorcarditis	Chordae Tendinae
o Hypertrophic cardiomyopathy	o Rupture (myocardial infarction)
	o Mitral Valve prolapse
	o Endocarditis
Mitral Annulus	o Rheumatic fever
o Calcification (rheumatic fever, chronic renal failure)	o Trauma
o Dilatation	

Table 3.1

What are some of the fundamental aspects of the pathophysiology of chronic mitral regurgitation?

- An abnormality in the anatomy or function of the valve will cause regurgitation that begins at the time of closure of the valve.
- The regurgitant volume (the amount of blood that enters the left atria from the ventricle during systole) will cause a number of other changes.

- The regurgitant volume depends on the following factors:
    - Size of the mitral valve orifice,
    - Heart rate
    - LV-LA pressure gradient during systole
    - Cardiac output
    - Afterload

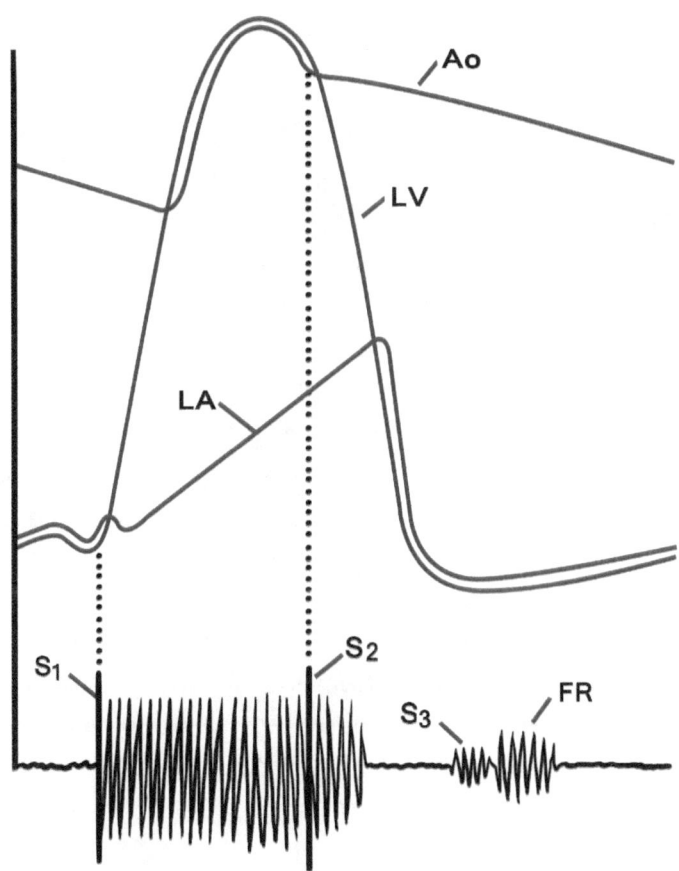

Fig 3.3. Schematic representations of LV and LA pressure, pressure gradient, and the murmurs observed. Systolic pressure gradient between ventricle and atria generates the systolic murmur. Increased diastolic flow across the valve caused by the increased atrial volume causes a diastolic murmur.

Regurgitant fraction (the ratio of regurgitant volume to end-diastolic volume) is an indication of the hemodynamic severity of the mitral regurgitation.

- ○ If less than 30%, patients are likely to be asymptomatic or mildly symptomatic.
- ○ If it is 30–60%, symptoms are moderate.
- ○ If greater than 60%, they will be very symptomatic.

Atrial compliance is important in the clinical presentations of mitral regurgitation.

- ○ In chronic mitral regurgitation, because of the gradual increase in the volume of the left atria, atrial pressure may remain closer to normal. A giant left atria is more often seen with severe chronic mitral regurgitation. Atrial compliance will increase as the atria dilates, as observed often in chronic regurgitation, and an initial moderate regurgitant volume will gradually stretch the atrial walls and increase atrial volume and compliance.
- ○ Patients with increased atrial compliance will have lower atrial pressures and often are free of symptoms for a long time. This is often seen in patients with chronic mitral regurgitation.
- ○ Patients with decreased atrial compliance, as seen in acute mitral regurgitation, will have high atrial pressures often causing acute pulmonary edema (see next case).

Other pathophysiological changes associated with mitral regurgitation include the following:

- ○ Increased left ventricular end-diastolic volume—the left ventricle has to provide both the

regurgitant volume as well as the forward stroke volume.
- Left ventricle dilatation progressively leads to left ventricular hypertrophy.
- The increase in LV volume will increase LV radius, and the results are as follows:
  - The increase of volume will lead increase contractility, according Frank-Starling Law. Clinically, this will manifest by a faster upstroke of arterial pulses and slight elevation of systolic pressure.
  - Left ventricular work will increase.
  - Ventricular wall stress will increase (to the fourth power of the ventricular radius), and this change influences subendocardial flow that may lead to subendocardial myocardial ischemia.
  - Increased volume has to return to the ventricle, and as a result, during rapid ventricular filling, the large volume can cause a brief diastolic murmur of low frequency.

The changes mentioned above can be translated into the pressure volume curve shown below.

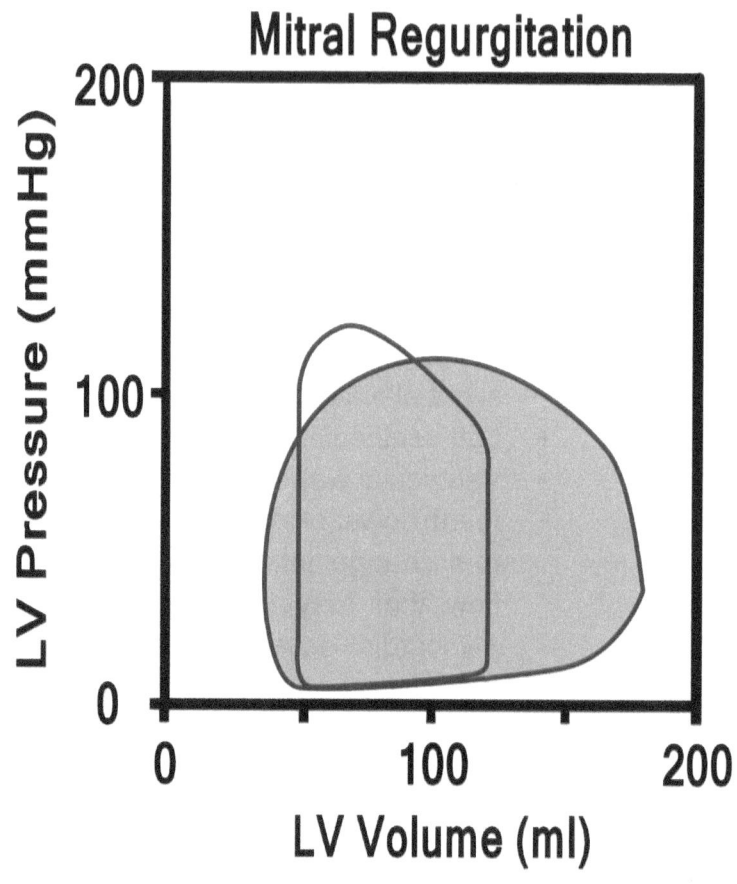

Fig 3.4. Pressure volume loop in chronic mitral regurgitation.

The volume of mitral regurgitation will be an interaction between preload (left atrial systolic pressure) and afterload systemic vascular resistance. From a practical and therapeutic perspective, decreasing afterload will facilitate forward flow and result in lowering regurgitation during systole. An increase in afterload will create greater resistance to forward flow and consequently increase regurgitant volume. For this reason, afterload reduction is commonly used to decrease the amount of mitral regurgitation and protect the left ventricle.

The severity of mitral regurgitation can be evaluated, primarily with the use of echocardiography and angiography.

PATHOPHYSIOLOGY AND PHYSICAL FINDINGS

- If LV hypertrophy is present, apical impulse may be prominent and displaced to the left axilla reflecting the increased volume and hypertrophy.
- Arterial pulses may have a faster upstroke as a result of increased contractility caused by the dilatation of the left ventricle.
- A murmur will appear in systole, starting during isovolumetric contraction, and will last as long there is a gradient of pressure between ventricle and atria. Because of the decreasing pressure gradient, the murmur may decrease in intensity toward the end of systole as seen in acute mitral regurgitation.
- The intensity and duration of the murmur may also be affected by certain maneuvers and drugs. For example:
    - Infusion of a drug that causes vasoconstriction will raise systolic pressure, increase the pressure gradient and the amount of regurgitant volume, and as a result, will increase the intensity of the murmur.
    - A vasodilator will lower systolic pressure, decrease the gradient and the regurgitant volume, and decrease both intensity and duration of the murmur.
- During rapid ventricular filling, the large volume returning from the left atria can cause a brief low-frequency diastolic murmur that will be heard in cases of large mitral regurgitation.

TREATMENT

Medical treatment is directed primarily to delay progression and protect the left ventricle. One of the methods is reduction of afterload through the use of drugs such ACE inhibitors that will lower peripheral vascular resistance and decrease the regurgitant volume. Prevention of subacute bacterial endocarditis is also an important consideration.

Treatment of mitral regurgitation is surgical with either replacement of the valve or repair of the leaflets. New noninvasive techniques allow both repair and replacement through cardiac catheterization with very promising results.

CASE 3 QUESTIONS

1. In a patient with chronic mitral regurgitation, left atrial pressure will be

    a. Probably normal
    b. Always lower than normal
    c. Always elevated
    d. Determined by atrial compliance

2. In a patient with moderate to severe mitral regurgitation, atrial fibrillation, and elevated left atrial pressure

    a. "y" descent will be slow
    b. "y" descent will be faster than normal
    c. "x" descent will be normal
    d. "x" descent will be slow

3. In chronic mitral regurgitation, left ventricular end-diastolic volume is

    a. Normal
    b. Decreased
    c. Increased
    d. Determined by atrial compliance

4. A drug that lowers peripheral vascular resistance will

    a. Decrease regurgitant volume
    b. Increase regurgitant volume
    c. Increase contractility
    d. Increase ventricular end-diastolic volume

5. A drug that increases peripheral resistance and elevates systolic pressure

    a. Will decrease the intensity of the murmur
    b. Will increase the intensity and duration of the murmur
    c. Has no effect on the murmur
    d. Will increase intensity of S1

6. In patients with chronic mitral regurgitation, the increase in systolic pressure may lead to subendocardial ischemia because

    a. Coronary disease will occur
    b. Increase in ventricular radius increases transmural pressure
    c. Concentric ventricular hypertrophy is common
    d. Left ventricular compliance is decreased

7. The murmur of mitral regurgitation

    a. Will begin during isovolumetric contraction
    b. Will begin when semilunar valves open
    c. Not be influenced by ventricular pressure
    d. Will have the same intensity throughout systole

CASE NO. 4: ACUTE MITRAL REGURGITATION

A fifty-two-year-old attorney goes to the emergency department complaining of acute constrictive precordial pain of 8/10 severity. He also complains of nausea and appears pale and diaphoretic. On examination, his blood pressure is 100/60, pulse 100x', respiration 20x'.

Physical examination is unremarkable except for modest obesity. Cardiovascular examination only demonstrated an S4 at the apex. No murmurs are present. Lungs are clear showing, no wheezing or rales.

The ECG demonstrates an acute inferior myocardial infarction.

He is admitted to the cardiac unit for further treatment.

Two hours later, a nurse reports that the patient has abruptly become short of breath and his blood pressure has dropped to 80/60 mm Hg. He is cold, clammy, and perspiring profusely.

Cardiac auscultation has changed, demonstrating a soft S1 and a grade 2/6 decrescendo pansystolic murmur that occupies only the early part of systole.

Lungs reveal bibasilar rales and diffuse wheezing.

Cardiac catheterization demonstrates acute mitral regurgitation and a marked hypokinetic area in the inferior wall.

Patient has undergone successful cardiac surgery.

DISCUSSION

Acute mitral regurgitation leads to acute hemodynamic complications and constitutes a cardiology emergency since it results in life-threatening acute hemodynamic changes. It often mandates emergency cardiac surgery.

The most common cause is an acute myocardial infarction with associated infarction of one of the papillary muscles. Acute bacterial endocarditis or rupture of a chordae tendineae can also cause acute mitral regurgitation.

What are the pathophysiological consequences of acute mitral regurgitation?

- The initial hemodynamic alteration is the development of a regurgitant volume from the left ventricle to left atria.
- As opposed to chronic mitral regurgitation (discussed earlier), the acute onset of mitral regurgitation cannot be immediately accompanied by adaptive and compensatory changes involving the left atria.
- The left atria has no time to stretch and dilate, resulting in the inability to increase left atrial volume, causing the rapid rise in atrial pressure. Pressure changes will be much greater than volume changes, and left atrial compliance decreases.
- The increase in left atrial pressure will result in an elevated "v" wave and a rapid "y" descent.
- Acutely cannot increase cardiac output, and the consequence is a decrease in stroke volume.
- The hemodynamic changes will have the following consequences:

    ○ *Elevation in pulmonary capillary pressure.* This will rapidly lead of fluid to transudate to the pulmonary alveoli causing pulmonary edema.

- *Hypotension and cardiogenic shock.* Initially, forward (or effective) stroke volume will decrease since total stroke volume has to divide itself between regurgitation volume to the left atria and effective stroke volume to the systemic circulation.
- The acutely decreased stroke volume causes low cardiac output and lower systemic pressure. Cardiogenic shock will follow.
- A secondary change is the decrease in end-systolic volume and a slight increase end-diastolic volume.

- As a result of the above, left ventricular pressure / volume curve will change, as shown below.
- The elevation of the left atrial pressure and elevated capillary pressure could lead to reactive pulmonary vasoconstriction and pulmonary hypertension.

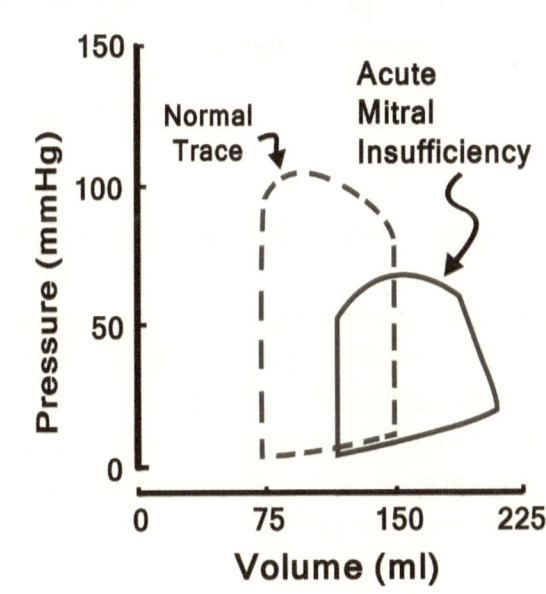

Fig. 4.2. Diagram of LV pressure-volume curve in acute mitral regurgitation.

As a result of the hemodynamic changes, the physical findings in acute mitral regurgitation will differ from those in chronic mitral regurgitation.

- The murmur will remain pansystolic (begins with isometric contraction) but will gradually decrease in intensity and often terminate early before the end of systole. The elevation of the "v" wave accompanied by the lower systemic pressure markedly decreases the pressure gradient between ventricular pressure and late systolic atrial pressure, resulting in late systolic termination of the murmur.

TREATMENT

The only possible treatment of acute mitral regurgitation is the repair of the valve apparatus or its replacement. If surgery must be performed in a patient with severe pulmonary edema, the mortality rate may be as high as 60%.

Supportive therapy while awaiting surgery should be directed.

- Decrease afterload while carefully monitoring systolic pressure.
- Decrease regurgitant volume to decrease left atrial pressure. Resulting drop in capillary pressure will decrease fluid flow to the alveoli.
- Support systemic pressure with drugs or intra-aortic balloon therapy (discussed in a subsequent case).

CASE 4 QUESTIONS

1. The most likely cause of the acute mitral regurgitation is

    a. Cardiomyopathy
    b. Papillary muscle infarction
    c. Myocardial rupture
    d. Pulmonary embolus

2. Acute mitral regurgitation will cause

    a. Decreased end-systolic volume
    b. Increased end-diastolic volume
    c. Increased stroke volume
    d. Increased afterload

3. Acute MR will cause

    a. Increase in left atrial volume
    b. Abnormal atrial pressure/volume curve
    c. Increased capillary oncotic pressure
    d. Decreased pulmonary capillary pressure

4. Acute MR can cause

    a. Arterial hypertension
    b. Arterial hypotension
    c. Increased cardiac output
    d. Decrease peripheral vascular resistance

5. In a patient with acute MR

    a. Total stroke volume will decrease
    b. Effective stroke volume will increase
    c. LV preload will decrease
    d. End-systolic volume will decrease

6. In a patient with acute MR, stroke volume is likely to decrease because of

    a. Decreased myocardial contractility
    b. Cardiogenic shock
    c. Mitral regurgitation volume
    d. Decreased preload

7. The reasons for his pulmonary edema is

    a. Cardiogenic shock
    b. Increased capillary oncotic pressure
    c. Increased left atrial pressure
    d. Pulmonary vasoconstriction

CASE NO. 5: MITRAL VALVE PROLAPSE

CP, a twenty-three-year-old graduate student, comes for a consultation, complaining of frequent palpitations. Her primary care physician had recognized a short systolic murmur and requested a consultation. During the interview, she denies any other cardiac symptoms. She is very active and exercises a lot without complaints.

Physical examination is unremarkable except for the cardiovascular system that revealed the following:

- No evidence of ventricular hypertrophy.
- Jugular and arterial pulses were normal.
- Auscultation revealed a normal S1 and S2. A midsystolic click was audible and followed by a late systolic murmur of mid to high frequency.

The ECG is normal.

DISCUSSION

The clinical presentation and physical findings support the diagnosis of mitral prolapse.

Mitral valve prolapse (MVP) is characterized by myxomatous degeneration of the mitral valve and the displacement of an abnormally thickened mitral valve leaflet into the left atrium during systole.

In severe cases of MVP, mitral regurgitation is present, and the risk of infective endocarditis is increased.

The echocardiogram is a valuable tool to evaluate this type of lesion and often shows protrusion of one of the leaflets into the left atria.

Minor MVP carries a low risk of complications, and regurgitation is minimal.

Patients with classic mitral valve prolapse have excess connective tissue that thickens the spongiosa and separates collagen bundles in the fibrosa of the valve. This is due to an excess of dermatan sulfate, a glycosaminoglycan. The leaflets and adjacent tissue are weakened, resulting in increased leaflet area and elongation of the chordae tendineae.

Elongation of the chordae tendineae often causes rupture, commonly to the chordae attached to the posterior leaflet. Advanced lesions—also commonly involving the posterior leaflet—lead to leaflet folding, inversion, and displacement toward the left atrium.

The murmur occurs late in systole and is usually preceded by a click triggered by tension on the valve apparatus. The murmur becomes louder on the standing position or during Valsalva, while squatting decreases the intensity.

TREATMENT

Individuals with mitral valve prolapse, particularly those without symptoms, often require no treatment.

Those with mitral valve prolapse and palpitations and chest pain may benefit from beta-blockers (e.g., propranolol). The pathophysiology of these symptoms is not clear.

In rare instances, when mitral valve prolapse is associated with severe mitral regurgitation, mitral valve repair or surgical replacement may be necessary.

Current ACC/AHA guidelines promote repair of mitral valve in patients before symptoms of heart failure develop.

Symptomatic patients, those with evidence of diminished left ventricular function or those with left ventricular dilatation, need more urgent attention.

Patients with prior stroke and/or atrial fibrillation may require blood thinners, such as aspirin or warfarin.

CASE 5 QUESTIONS

1. The prevalence of mitral prolapse is

    a. 1% of the population
    b. 2% of the population
    c. 5% of the population
    d. 10% of the population

2. The murmur of mitral prolapse is accentuated by

    a. Squatting
    b. Valsalva
    c. Inspiration
    d. Expiration

3. One the following conditions is associated with MVP

    a. Tetralogy of Fallot
    b. Ehler-Danlos syndrome
    c. Aortic coarctation
    d. Obesity

4. Decreased end-diastolic volume

    a. Decreases intensity of the MVP murmur
    b. Increases intensity of MVP murmur
    c. Does not change intensity of the murmur
    d. Causes the click to disappear

5. One of the following is correct:

    a. In MVP, chordae tendinae are shortened
    b. Patients with MVP have increased connective tissue in leaflets
    c. Have decreased content of dermatan sulfate in the valve
    d. The anterior leaflet is the one mostly affected

CASE NO. 6: TRICUSPID REGURGITATION

A twenty-three-year-old male presents to the ED complaining of high fever and chills of two days' duration. In addition, he feels weak and has lost some weight in the last two weeks. He states that he has been addicted to heroin for more than one year and injects himself at least twice a day with his own poorly sterilized needle and syringe.

In the ED, he appears chronically ill with a temperature of 38.8 degrees centigrade. Pulse is 105 per minute and respiration 18x'.

Examination reveals multiple needle marks in the upper and lower extremities.

Cardiovascular examination shows the following:

- Slightly distended jugular veins with a visible large "v" wave and a rapid "y" descent.
- Precordial palpation reveals no ventricular hypertrophy.
- Arterial pulses are normal.
- On auscultation,
    - First and second heart sounds were normal.
    - A soft, mid-frequency decrescendo pansystolic grade 2/6 murmur is best heard over the left fourth intercostal space. The murmur distinctly increases during inspiration.
    - A third heart sound is audible over the tricuspid area.

Remaining of the physical examination is unremarkable.

The patient is admitted for diagnosis and treatment of acute bacterial endocarditis. An echocardiogram was obtained.

The patient was admitted and started on antibiotic therapy and recovered well.

DISCUSSION

The history of longstanding heroin addiction, coupled with multiple needle marks, the use of poorly sterilized needles, high fever, and a systolic murmur that increases with inspiration made clinicians suspect tricuspid bacterial endocarditis. The diagnosis was confirmed with several blood cultures that grew staphylococcus and by the echocardiogram that showed the regurgitation and a vegetation in the tricuspid valve.

Tricuspid regurgitation can be either acute or chronic. Acute is most often the consequence of bacterial endocarditis, while chronic is most often the consequence of chronic right heart failure and, less commonly, the consequence of rheumatic fever. Other potential causes of tricuspid regurgitation include

- Ebstein anomaly,
- tricuspid valve prolapse,
- carcinoid,
- papillary muscle dysfunction,
- trauma,
- connective-tissue diseases, and
- medications.

Factors that can contribute to infection of the valve, in addition to IV drug abuse, include infected indwelling catheters, extensive burns, and immune deficiency. The clinical presentation of acute tricuspid endocarditis is often that of pneumonia from septic pulmonary emboli rather than CHF. Heart murmurs are frequently absent or very soft systolic murmurs, and blood cultures may be negative. Annular abscesses are not uncommon.

THE PATHOPHYSIOLOGICAL CHANGES IN TRICUSPID REGURGITATION

- Inspiratory increase of the regurgitant volume. The increase in venous return during inspiration increases right ventricular volume and increases regurgitant volume.
- Dilation of the right ventricle, resulting from regurgitation across the valve.
- Derangement of the normal anatomy and mechanics of the tricuspid valve and the papillary muscles, preventing proper function.
- The RV adapts better to volume overload than to pressure overload and may tolerate volume overload without a significant decrease in RV systolic function. Long-standing volume overload may lead to an increase in morbidity and mortality.
- Right ventricular diastolic dysfunction impairs RV filling and increases diastolic volume, RV pressures, and right atrial pressures.
- The increase in RV volume may lead to fluid retention and liver congestion.
- RV failure may also increase tricuspid regurgitation, which may further aggravate RV volume overload and decrease cardiac output.

How does the pathophysiology affect the physical findings?

- All right-sided murmur should increase with inspiration. The exception to this practical rule is with very advanced right ventricular failure with major ventricular dilatation that limits any further increase in inspiratory right ventricular volume.

- The few physical findings associated with acute TR are functions of the compliance of the right atrium. The right atrium is unable to dilate acutely, and the result is a marked elevation of the "v" wave. In addition, RV pressure is most likely normal or minimally elevated. As a result of both factors, the late systolic pressure gradient between the RV pressure and the "v wave" is minimal, and the murmur would then markedly decrease its intensity or will terminate.
- The murmur is soft and of mid frequency. Since right ventricular pressure is not very elevated, the ventricular/atrial pressure gradient is small.
- Chronically, tricuspid regurgitation leads to right-sided congestive heart failure (CHF). This manifests as hepatic congestion, peripheral edema, and ascites.
- Hepatic congestion often causes a pulsatile liver, ascites, and peripheral edema, and in more advanced cases, it can lead to hepatic cirrhosis.

As shown by this case, endocarditis is an important cause of tricuspid regurgitation.

Chronic TR is the result of right ventricular dilatation of any cause. Such dilatation is most often the result of left heart failure (of any cause) or pulmonary hypertension.

TREATMENT

Medical treatment for acute endocarditis caused by bacterial infection requires identification of the organism. The two more common are *Staphylococcus aureus* and *Pseudomonas aeruginosa*.

The need for valve replacement is rather uncommon, and implantation of a ring to narrow the valve orifice is sometimes indicated.

CASE 6 QUESTIONS

1. In a patient with large tricuspid regurgitation, failure of the murmur to increase with inspiration usually indicates

    a. Increased stroke volume
    b. Decreased ventricular compliance
    c. Severe right heart failure
    d. Associated left heart failure

2. The right ventricle

    a. Tolerates pressure overload better
    b. Tolerate volume overload better
    c. Systolic function will not be affected by heart failure
    d. Diastolic RV dysfunction will not increase end-diastolic RV pressure

3. Tricuspid regurgitation causes

    a. Increased "a" wave
    b. Increased "x" descent
    c. Faster "y" descent
    d. Elevated RV systolic pressure

4. In a patient with acute severe TR

    a. Atrial compliance is increased
    b. Atrial compliance is decreased
    c. Ventricular compliance is always increased
    d. RV stroke volume will decrease

CASE NO. 7: VALVULAR AORTIC STENOSIS

Mr. JJ is a seventy-two-year-old retired college professor that was referred for evaluation of a recent fainting episode and a heart murmur. The fainting episode happened on a hot summer day and during a brisk walk. The loss of consciousness lasted only a few seconds. He recovered quickly and refused to be taken to the hospital. He denied any similar episodes in the past. He reported an active life, walked one and a half miles every day without shortness of breath or chest pain. Previous examinations had revealed a loud ejection systolic murmur.

Physical examination by the cardiologist revealed the following:

- Normal JVP
- Slow upstroke of the arterial pulses
- All peripheral pulses present
- Sustained nondisplaced apical impulse
- Normal S1, soft aortic component of S2, S4 at the apex, harsh grade 4/6 ejection systolic murmur best heard on the aortic area radiating to the neck with maximal intensity in mid to late systole

DISCUSSION

The clinical findings suggest aortic stenosis, manifested by the fainting episode, the presence of ventricular hypertrophy, the slow rising arterial pulses, and the loud ejection murmur.

Aortic stenosis creates an obstruction to the left ventricular systolic emptying. The obstruction can be located at

- the valve (secondary to abnormalities in leaflet anatomy),

- above the valve (supravalvular aortic stenosis, congenital),
- below the valve (subvalvular stenosis, congenital),
- cardiac muscle (obstructive cardiomyopathy).

Patients with a left ventricular obstruction can also be subdivided into the following:

- *Fixed obstruction.* The anatomical lesion (valvular, supravalvular, or subvalvular) is fixed throughout systole, and the level of obstruction remains unchanged. Valvular aortic stenosis is the classical example of fixed orifice obstruction since the valve with fused cusps will have a narrowed orifice that will remain of the same size throughout the cardiac cycle.

Valvular aortic stenosis is the most common of all types of LV outflow obstruction.

In patients younger than seventy years of age, the cause is likely as follows:

- **Bicuspid aortic valve............................ 50%**
- Postinflammatory (i.e., rheumatic) 25%
- Degenerative.. 18%
- Other... 7%

In patients older than seventy years of age, the cause is likely as follows:

- **Degenerative...................................... 48%**
- Bicuspid aortic valve............................ 27%
- Postinflammatory................................. 23%
- Other... 2%

Valvular aortic stenosis is either the result of previous rheumatic fever or is a congenital lesion, commonly a bicuspid valve.

A **bicuspid aortic valve** is a congenital anomaly sometimes (25%) associated with aortic regurgitation. It results from the fusion of two leaflets and affects approximately 1.2% of adults. One of the most notable associations with bicuspid aortic valve is the tendency for these patients to present with ascending aortic aneurysmal lesions. The extracellular matrix of the aorta in patients with a bicuspid valve shows marked deviations from that of the normal tricuspid aortic valve. It is currently believed that an increase in the ratio of MMP2 (matrix metalloproteinases 2) to TIMP1 (tissue inhibitor metalloproteinases 1) may be responsible for the abnormalities of the valve matrix, and that leads to aortic dissection and aneurysm.

Aortic valve sclerosis (AVS) was considered a normal degenerative process associated with aging. The soft basal ejection murmur of aortic sclerosis was generally regarded to have little clinical significance. Aortic valve sclerosis has emerged as a biomarker for cardiovascular risk and ultimately can lead to aortic stenosis.

- *Variable obstruction.* Muscular (obstructive cardiomyopathy) where an abnormality in the cardiac muscle causes the obstruction to flow. Changes in contractility will affect the degree of obstruction. Obstructive cardiomyopathy is the classic entity where the size of the left ventricular outflow varies during the cardiac cycle. It will be reviewed in a subsequent case.

The pathophysiology of left ventricular outflow obstruction is as follows:

- The stenosis slows and delays emptying of the left ventricle. It takes longer for the stroke volume to leave the ventricular chamber.
- Systole is longer, and the closure of the aortic valve is delayed. The severity of the obstruction will influence the delay.

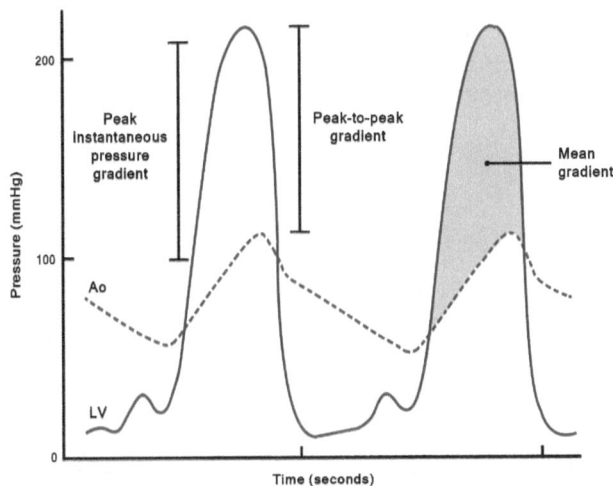

Fig. 7.2. Schematic representation of the pressure gradient between the left ventricle and the ascending aorta.

The changes in pressure (gradient) and flow generate turbulence as blood enters to the ascending aorta. The turbulence causes a murmur in systole and often a palpable thrill commonly in the right second intercostal space.

- The turbulence alters the distribution of jet forces. Forces will gradually impact the aortic wall and eventually result in dilatation of the ascending aorta (post stenotic dilatation).

Hemodynamics of a Stenosis

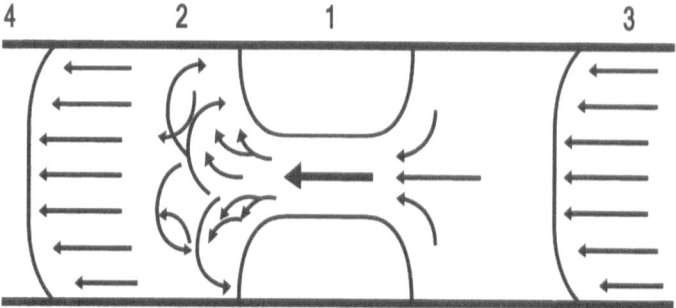

Zone 1 - Abrupt increase in velocity at PMS
Zone 2 - Abrupt decrease in velocity with turbulence
Zone 3 - Evidence of increased downstream resistancev
Zone 4 - Permanent energy losses (pressure), delayed systolic upstroke ("tardus parcus" waveform)

Fig. 7.3. *Left.* Diagrammatic representation of the hemodynamic of aortic stenosis and the creation of turbulent flow across the obstruction.

* The turbulence will propagate through the ascending aorta and preferentially to the right carotid artery because of the continuity of flow. This explains why the aortic stenosis murmur is best heard to the right carotid. In addition, the lower diastolic arterial pressure also decreases the leaflet mobility.

* The increased duration of left ventricular systole delays closure of the aortic valve.

* The obstruction at the valve slows down the velocity of ejection.

* The increased left ventricular pressure resulting from increased impedance due to the obstruction leads to left ventricular hypertrophy, concentric in nature. This in turn will

- decrease left ventricular compliance,

- increase left ventricular end-diastolic pressure, and

- decrease left ventricular end-systolic volume.

* The increased ventricular thickness, the elevated end-diastolic pressure, and the decreased flow velocity and flow will lead to subendocardial ischemia.

All these hemodynamic changes will be shown in the left ventricular pressure volume curve.

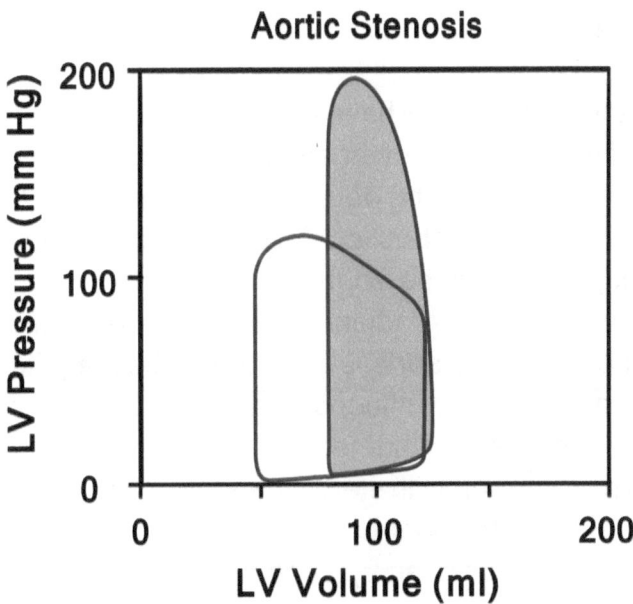

Fig. 7.4. Pressure volume curve in aortic stenosis.

The pathophysiology of the lesion influences the physical findings.

- The apical impulse is sustained and is larger, and a presystolic impulse is often felt, coinciding with an S4 and caused by decreased compliance of the ventricle.
- An ejection click can be audible if the leaflets retain mobility.
- Intensity of the aortic component can decrease if the leaflet mobility is impaired.
- Aortic component of S2 is delayed. Obstruction delays emptying and prolongs systole.
- In cases of severe aortic stenosis, aortic closure may occur after pulmonic closure resulting in *paradoxical splitting of the second heart sound,* since RV systole is unaffected during inspiration and it may superimpose valve closure with the aortic closure. During expiration, the normal separation between the two components can be reversed.
- Arterial pulses will have slower upstroke. The obstruction will generate a slower emptying of the left ventricle and will slow down the development of pressure (and flow) beyond the obstruction. This will slow down the building of pressure in the aorta.
- The pressure gradient between the left ventricle and the ascending aorta is generated. The magnitude of the gradient will be influenced by the severity of the lesion and the stroke volume.
- The murmur will start when the valve opens, after isovolumetric contraction.
- The murmur is an *ejection* type, and its timing during systole will be dependent on the severity of the lesion. The more severe the stenosis, the longer the murmur and the later it will reach maximum intensity. The

intensity, however, will be influenced not only by the severity of the lesion but also by the stroke volume.

In the natural history of aortic stenosis, the physiological changes may lead to the following symptoms:

- *Angina pectoris.* Angina occurs when there is an abnormal supply/demand relationship. This is caused by the following:
    - The increased cardiac mass, resulting from the concentric hypertrophy, increases O_2 demand.
    - Coronary flow decreases because of the lowering of aortic pressure.
    - The turbulence created leads to abnormal distribution of flow. These factors, together with decreases in stroke volume, decrease flow into the coronaries.
- *Sudden death / syncope.* Several factors are implicated:
    - The myocardial ischemia mentioned above can trigger ventricular arrhythmias.
    - Hypotensive episode, secondary to exercise, may trigger increased ischemia and result in sudden death.
- *Heart failure.* The decreased compliance elevates end-diastolic pressure and may lead to pulmonary edema. In addition, the hypertrophy as well as the underlying ischemia may affect myocardial function and lead to heart failure.

When these symptoms develop, prognosis is guarded, and in many cases, death may occur in a brief period of time. The approximate interval between the onset of symptoms and death are as follows:

Heart failure... 1–2 years

Syncope............3 years

Angina...............5 years

Mortality rate after the onset of symptoms:

- 25% at 1 year
- 50% at 2 years

Echocardiography is a very useful technology to evaluate aortic stenosis and to determine its severity facilitating some prognostic conclusions, as shown in the following table from the American Heart Association and American College of Cardiology.

Classification of AS severity

(ᵃESC & ᵇAHA/ACC Guidelines)

	Aortic Sclerosis	Mild	Moderate	Severe
Aortic jet velocity (m/s)	2.5 m/s	2.6 – 2.9	3.0 – 4	> 4
Mean gradient (mm Hg)		< 20 (<30)	20 – 40 (30 – 50a)	> 40
AVA (cm²)		> 1.5	1.0 – 1.5	< 1.0
Indexed AVA (cm²/m²)		> 0.85	0.60 – 0.85	< 0.6
Velocity ratio		> 0.50	0.25 – 0.50	< 0.25

Table 7.2

TREATMENT

Treatment requires a surgical procedure with replacement or repair of the aortic valve. If valvular replacement is indicated, the type of valve used will be determined by the age of the patient.

The current approaches are as follows:

VALVE REPLACEMENT

There are different types of artificial valve. Biological valves should be used in older patients since they tend to degrade after ten years and may require a new replacement. All these valves require the patient to be anticoagulated.

TRANSAORTIC VALVE REPLACEMENT

New techniques allow replacement without need of a thoracotomy.

Replacement of the aortic valve percutaneously through the femoral artery is now an accepted procedure, and the device is shown below. This type or procedure is preferred at present for older very symptomatic individuals that represent a very high surgical risk.

There is no medical treatment available; although some studies reported that cholesterol-lowering agents may help in slowing down the sclerotic progression.

CASE 7 QUESTIONS

1. In a patient with severe aortic stenosis, left ventricular compliance is

    a. Decreased
    b. Increased
    c. Normal
    d. Unchanged

2. In a patient with severe aortic stenosis, peak pressure gradient across the aortic valve will be greatest during

    a. Late systole
    b. Early systole
    c. Not influenced by severity
    d. Determined by duration of diastole

3. In a patient with severe aortic stenosis, the murmur loses intensity if

    a. Patient is febrile
    b. Patient exercises
    c. Stroke volume is low
    d. End-diastolic volume is high

4. In a patient with severe aortic stenosis, paradoxical S2 may happen because of

    a. Early pulmonary valve closure
    b. Prolonged ejection time
    c. Decreased contractility
    d. Increased compliance

5. In a patient with aortic stenosis, a pressure/volume loop will demonstrate

    a. Increased stroke volume
    b. Elevated end-diastolic pressure
    c. Increased end-diastolic volume
    d. Decreased LV pressure

6. The cause of an ejection click is

    a. Calcified valve
    b. Mobile but fused leaflets
    c. Decreased contractility
    d. Normal stroke volume

CASE NO. 8: CHRONIC AORTIC REGURGITATION

An eighteen-year-old college student is referred for consultation before receiving a basketball scholarship. He reports being in excellent health and in excellent physical condition, having trained and competed in basketball during his high school years. Having detected a murmur, the school physician decided he needed a cardiovascular evaluation.

On physical examination, he was six feet six inches tall and weighs 130 pounds. General examination reveals no abnormalities, although he appears to have slightly longer upper extremities. Physical examination is unremarkable except for the cardiovascular system reported as follows:

- BP = 155/60, P = 60x', R = 16x'
- Normal jugular venous pulses.
- Arterial pulses are bounding and have a very rapid usptroke.
- Palpation of the precordium shows an apical impulse diffused and slightly displaced laterally.

On auscultation, first-heard sound is soft. Aortic component of the second heart sound is louder than normal. A grade 2/6 ejection systolic murmur is heard over the aortic area, and a grade 2/6, high-frequency, blowing, decrescendo diastolic murmur is heard over the aortic area radiating along both sides of the sternum. A low-frequency diastolic murmur is detected at the apex, starting after a soft third heart sound.

Remaining of the physical examination is unremarkable.

Because of his height and weight and general physical charcteristics, the cardiologist indicates that aortic regurgitation, probably secondary to Marfan syndrome, is very likely. He recommends that he and siblings undergo genetic testing.

DISCUSSION

Aortic regurgitation can be caused by a large number of diseases as listed below:

- *Abnormalities of the aortic valve*
    - Bicuspid aortic valve
    - Rheumatic fever
    - Infective endocarditis
    - Collagen vascular diseases
    - Degenerative aortic valve diseases
    - Traumatic postsurgical

- *Abnormalities of the ascending aorta*
    - Hypertension
    - Marfan syndrome
    - Cystic medial necrosis
    - Syphilitic aortitis
    - Giant cell arteritis
    - Ankylosing spondylitis

The case under discussion suggests Marfan syndrome, a genetic disorder, autosomal dominant. In 75% of patients, the condition is inherited from a parent, while 25% of the time, it is a new mutation. The genetic anomaly involves a mutation to the gene *FBN1* on chromosome 15, resulting in abnormal connective tissue. The most serious complications involve the heart and with an increased risk of mitral valve prolapse and aortic aneurysm. Aortic regurgitation is common.

The prevalence of AR, of any etiology or severity, ranges from 2–30%. The prevalence of severe AR is less than 1% in the general population.

- Prevalence of AR increases with age.
- Severity of the disease affects survival:

- Patients with significant aortic regurgitation survive five years after the diagnosis.
- Around 50% survive for ten years.
- Around 85% of patients with mild to moderate regurgitation survive ten years.
- Onset of heart failure has a survival of less than two years.

What are the pathophysiological changes in chronic AR?

The pathophysiology starts when the aortic valve becomes incompetent and is unable to close properly. Part of the stroke volume then is returned to the left ventricle during diastole.

- As a result of the regurgitant volume, the end-diastolic volume increases.
- Volume overload leads to compensatory changes that include the following:
  - LV enlargement
  - LV eccentric hypertrophy
  - LV dilation, resulting in longer myocardial fibers
  - Compliance of the dilated LV increases
- Stroke volume increases since it must include the amount that will reenter the left ventricle to maintain a normal cardiac output.
- The increased LV volume and consequent dilatation results in increased wall tension and stress (Laplace's law).
- LV ejection fraction (EF) is normal or increased (due to the increased preload and the Frank-Starling mechanism).

- LV end-systolic volume rises in the late stages of chronic AR and is a sensitive indicator of progressive myocardial dysfunction.
- In late stages, LV reaches its maximum diameter, and end-diastolic pressure begins to rise, resulting in dyspnea.
- The LV gradually evolves from its normal elliptical configuration to a more spherical one.

The pressure-volume curve will gradually change as a consequence of the dilatation with gradual pressure/volume changes discussed above.

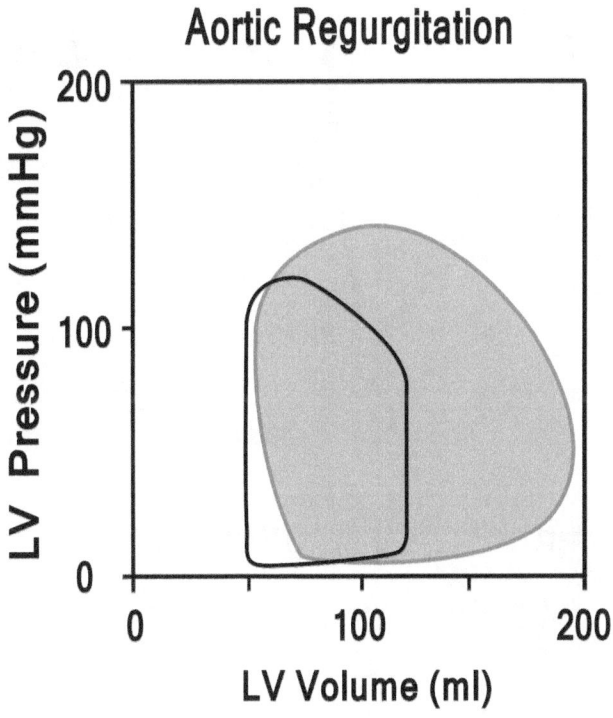

Fig. 8.1. Pressure volume loop in chronic aortic regurgitation.

- Myocardial ischemia may develop. It results from decreased coronary perfusion gradients resulting from the lower aortic diastolic pressure. In addition, the increased LV mass influences the perfusion ratio. Subendocardial ischemia, necrosis, and apoptosis may occur.

A low diastolic pressure is a good estimate of the severity. It is commonly expressed as the aortic regurgitation index, calculated as shown below:

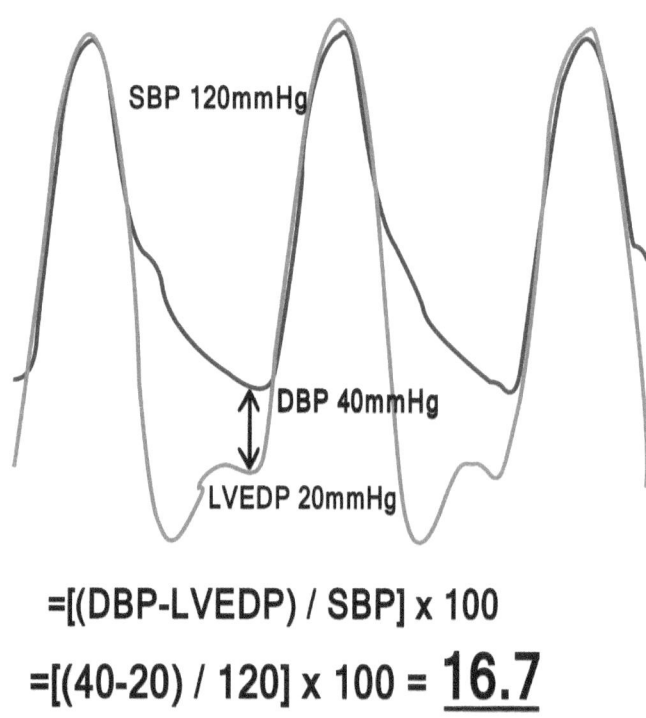

Fig. 8.2. Calculation of AR index. DBP = diastolic blood pressure. LVEDP = left ventricular diastolic pressure. SBP = systolic blood pressure.

As a result of the physiological changes, a physical examination may reveal the following:

- Displaced LV impulse from the dilatation of the LV
- Visible pulsations in places such as the uvula, the capillary bed, etc. resulting from the increased pulse pressure. This happens in more severe aortic regurgitation.
- Very wide pulse pressure sometimes manifested by pulsations of the head (head bobbing).
- An ejection murmur is often heard, resulting from turbulence generated by the increased stroke volume.
- A diastolic murmur—the murmur starts immediately after closure of aortic valve and is usually of high frequency because of the large pressure gradient between ascending aorta and LV during diastole.
- As the pressure gradient gradually decreases during diastole, the murmur decreases in intensity in late diastole.
- The regurgitant jet, as it enters the LV outflow tract, will make contact with the anterior leaflet of the mitral valve, resulting in both early closure and fluttering of the mitral valve. These cause a low-frequency diastolic murmur (Austin Flint murmur).

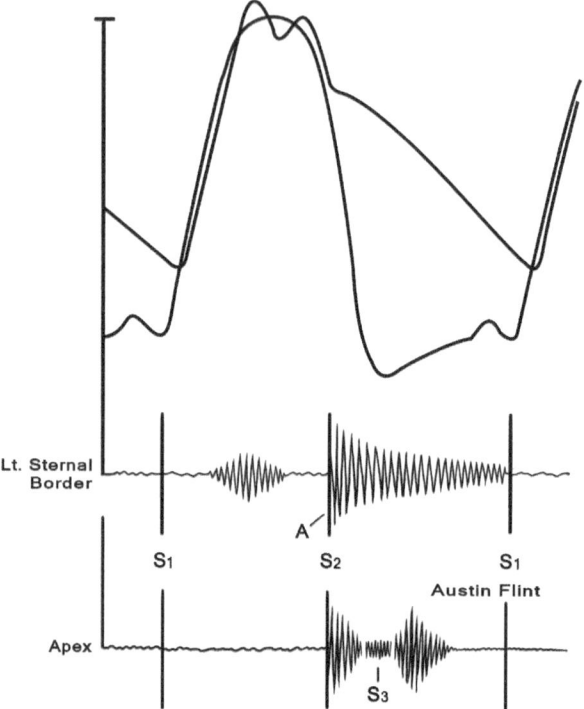

Fig. 8.3. Diagrammatic representation of pressures and murmurs in AR.

- The ejection murmur must be distinguished from associated aortic stenosis.

These auscultatory findings are illustrated above.

TREATMENT

As indicated above, chronic AR is usually associated with good survival, and the clinical approach should be very conservative with periodic surveillance. Echocardiography is a good test to follow, not only for the amount of regurgitant volume but also the ventricular size.

Medical treatment is directed to the protection of the left ventricle by decreasing afterload that decreases peripheral resistance and also decreases the regurgitant volume.

When surgery becomes indicated, valve replacement is the alternative, and in recent years, transaortic percutaneous replacement has gained acceptance, especially in elderly or high surgical risks population.

CASE 8 QUESTIONS

1. In a patient with chronic aortic regurgitation, end-diastolic volume is

    a. Normal
    b. Decreased
    c. Increased
    d. Unchanged

2. In chornic AR, myocardial oxygen consumption is

    a. Decreased
    b. Increased
    c. Normal
    d. Not influenced by the AR

3. In chronic aortic regurgitation, LV stroke work is increased because

    a. End diastolic volume in increased
    b. Diastolic arterial presure is increased
    c. Systolic arterial pressure is increased
    d. End-diastolic pressure is increased

4. In chronic AR, myocardial contractility is

    a. Decreased
    b. Normal
    c. Increased
    d. Unchanged

5. The explanation for the increase in contractility is

    a. Increased systolic pressure
    b. Decreased diastolic pressure

c. Increased end-diastolic volume
   d. Increased stroke colume

6. The Austin Flynn murmur

   a. Is caused by early closure of the mitral valve
   b. Is seen in all cases of AR
   c. Is midsystolic
   d. Is high frequency

CASE NO. 9: ACUTE AORTIC REGURGITATION

Mrs. AA, a sixty-two-year-old man, arrived to the ED complaining of excruciating chest pain that started approximately fifteen minutes prior to arrival. In this period of time, the pain migrated to the back and has not decreased in intensity.

Family reported a longstanding history of essential hypertension, poorly controlled. No murmurs were reported previously.

Upon arrival, BP was 190/80 mm Hg, pulse was 100x', and respiration 20x'.

A limited cardiovascular examination was performed that revealed a grade 2/6 election systolic murmur and a grade 2/6 diastolic murmur, both heard at the second right intercostal space.

Because of the severity of the symptoms, the patient was administered two milligrams of morphine. She was transported to radiology where a CT of the chest was performed.

This course of action was justified because the intensity and location of the pain and the presence of a new diastolic aortic murmur strongly suggested an acute aortic dissection in progress. The CT scan demonstrated aortic dissection with a distinct false lumen.

The patient was immediately started on beta-blockers intravenously, and a thoracic surgeon was consulted.

DISCUSSION

This patient had the classical presentation of aortic dissection—excruciating chest pain that migrated and radiated to the back, a new murmur of aortic regurgitation, and a history of hypertension.

Aortic dissection is one of the causes of acute aortic regurgitation resulting from an acute disruption of the aortic valve support by the retrograde hematoma in the media of the ascending aorta. This hematoma may also rupture in the pericardium with an often fatal outcome.

The majority of aortic dissections begin in the ascending aorta and will extend to the descending aorta (60%). Dissection may be limited to the ascending aorta (15%) or to the descending aorta (25%).

The prevalence of dissection is 2 per 100,000 and represents the most common emergency involving the aorta. It is twice as common as rupture of the abdominal aorta.

Mortality associated to acute dissection is

- 50% in the first twenty-four hours and
- 75% in the first week.

The disease is a catastrophic emergency—40% do not reach a hospital on time. Of the remainder, even after the correct diagnosis is made, 5–20% die during surgery or in the immediate postoperative period.

With aggressive treatment, thirty-day survival of those correctly diagnosed may be as high as 90%.

Other causes of acute aortic regurgitation are as follows:

- Iatrogenic dissection
- Infective endocarditis
- Collagen vascular diseases
- Degenerative aortic valve disease
- Traumatic
- Postsurgical
- Abnormalities of the ascending aorta
    - Longstanding, uncontrolled hypertension
    - Marfan syndrome

What are the pathophysiological changes associated with acute aortic regurgitation?

The acute onset of a regurgitant volume, without time for any adaptive changes in the left ventricle, will lead to the following:

- Acute left ventricular overload resulting from the acute onset of a regurgitant volume.
- As a result to increase acutely is volume capacity
- With the change in ventricular compliance, LV end-diastolic pressure increases and may cause pulmonary edema.
- Stroke volume decreases because of the volume re-entering the LV decreases the remaining stroke volume
- The hemodynamic changes described above lowers systolic blood pressure often causing shock.
- Peripheral vascular resistance increases as opposed to what happens in chronic aortic regurgitation.
- Increased end-diastolic pressure increases wall stress and causes subendocardial ischemia.

The pressure volume curve shows the acute hemodynamic changes.

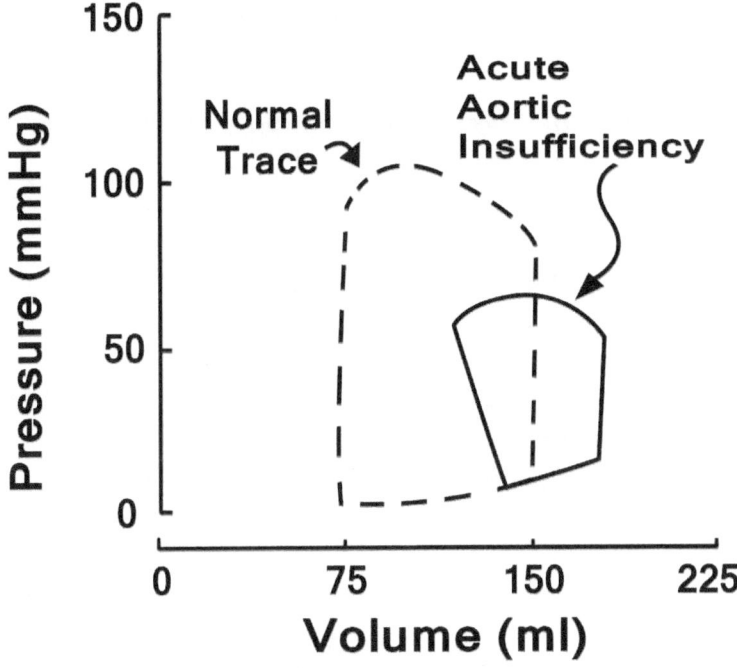

Fig. 9.2. Pressure-volume diagram in acute aortic regurgitation.

The physiological changes result in the following physical findings:

- Lower systolic pressure.
- Decreased intensity of S1.
- Diastolic murmur of recent onset.
- Murmur occupies only the initial part of diastole and quickly decreases since LV and aortic pressure rapidly equalize.

TREATMENT

Acute aortic regurgitation constitutes a surgical emergency and causes very unstable hemodynamics.

Medical treatment should be directed at preparing the patient for surgery, focusing on

- maximizing cardiac output,
- minimizing regurgitant volume, and
- reducing pulmonary venous congestion.

Reduction of afterload in a manner that maintains blood pressure and cardiac output should be the goal of initial therapy. Intravenous infusion of nitroprusside constitutes the best approach.

Surgical approach must be influenced by the etiology. Aortic valve repair or replacement must be decided. Transcatheter aortic valve replacement (TAVR) has emerged as an important therapy for aortic stenosis and is being evaluated for aortic regurgitation, but not enough data is available for cases of acute aortic dissection.

CASE 9 QUESTIONS

1. In acute aortic regurgitation, left ventricular end-diastolic volume is always increased

    a. True
    b. False

2. One of the following can be a cause of acute aortic regurgitation:

    a. Syphilis
    b. Spondyloarthrosis
    c. Endocarditis
    d. Rheumatic fever

3. One of the following occurs often in acute aortic regurgitation

    a. RV hypertrophy
    b. Low end-diastolic pressure
    c. Hypotension
    d. High arterial pressure

4. Aortic dissection involving the descending aorta

    a. Often involves the pericardium
    b. Should be treated medically
    c. Has a higher mortality rate than ascending dissection

CORONARY DISEASE

MYOCARDIAL ISCHEMIA

CASE NO 10: STABLE ANGINA PECTORIS

A sixty-two-year-old male is referred to a cardiologist to evaluate episodes of exercise-induced chest pain.

The patient reports that for the last three months, whenever he engages in a strenuous physical activity, he notices the onset of chest pain, often located in the pectoral region, radiates to the neck and jaw, and often accompanied by perspiration. He describes the pain as if someone is sitting on his chest and forces him to stop. The pain promptly subsides when he stops exercising. He never had pain at night or while resting. He has decreased his level of activity, and with mild activities, he has had no episodes of pain.

He had not consulted a physician until recently, and he was referred to a cardiologist for further evaluation and treatment.

He denies any family history of heart disease or any history of diabetes or hypertension.

On previous examinations, he was informed that his blood sugar was elevated and that he was obese for his age, height, and weight. He was advised to lose weight and engage in some regular physical activity but did not comply with the physician's recommendation.

On physical examination, the following is noted:

- Height 5'10", weight 220 lbs.
- Pulse rate is 78x' and blood pressure 160/90 mm Hg.
- Physical examination is essentially unremarkable except for a forty-two-inch waist compared to a chest circumference of thirty-eight inches.
- All peripheral pulses are present and normal.

His resting ECG was normal.

DISCUSSION

The clinical presentation is highly suggestive of angina pectoris. His history of untreated diabetes plus his obesity and elevated blood pressure make coronary artery disease the most likely diagnosis to be pursued for any patient with exercise-induced chest pain.

What are the probabilities of this being coronary disease? This depends on the individual's gender, age, and state of health. For example:

- Probability of CAD is very high (>90%) in a sixty-five-year-old obese male with history of type II diabetes mellitus and uncontrolled essential hypertension.

- Probability of CAD in a thirty-year-old menstruating female with no other risk factors is very low (+/-5%).

Evaluation of an individual risk must take into account the pretest likelihood of disease for that individual. This is illustrated in table 10.1. Based on this information, the diagnostic approach should be tailored.

PRE-TEST LIKELIHOOD OF CORONARY DISEASE

IN SYMPTOMATIC PATIENTS

ACCORDING TO AGE AND SEX

AJC 2007; 50.2064.74

AGE	NON ANGINAL		ATYPICAL ANGINAL		TYPICAL ANGINA	
	MEN	WOMEN	MEN	WOMEN	MEN	WOMEN
30 – 39	4	2	32	12	78	36
40 – 49	13	3	51	22	87	55
50 – 59	20	7	65	31	93	73
60 – 69	27	14	72	51	94	86

Table 10.1

Based on this information, the diagnosis of coronary artery disease should be pursued since the pretest likelihood of having coronary disease is greater than 90%.

How does the pain originate, and what are the pathways for pain? Manifestation in a patient with angina pectoris?

The onset of ischemic chest pain is correlated with the activation of an anaerobic metabolic pathway. It will be accompanied by the release in the coronary circulation of lactate as well as serotonin, bradykinin, histamine, and especially adenosine. The results are as follows:

- Degradation of ATP circulating at the extracellular level.
- Receptor stimulation of nerve endings.
- The nerve ending that receive the signals corresponds to spinal nerves 1–4.
- The signal then follows an upward path through the thalamus and spinal cords and, from there, to the cerebral cortex.
- Peculiarities of anatomical distribution of the nerve plexuses explain why the most common clinical forms of manifestation of chest pain have topographies at the chest, neck, shoulder, or left arm level.

What are some of the physiological changes associated with myocardial ischemia?

Under normal circumstances, myocardial metabolism is aerobic, and there is a constant balance between O_2 demand and supply. Whenever an individual increases demand of O_2, the myocardium must be supplied by an increase in oxygen to maintain the balance between myocardial oxygen demand and myocardial oxygen supply. This happens through increased coronary flow.

In a normal person, coronary blood flow can increase several folds and is unlikely for the myocardium to start operating in an anaerobic manner. Contrary, in a patient like the one we are discussing, coronary flow cannot increase enough to meet the needs, resulting in myocardial ischemia and angina pectoris.

Myocardial ischemia will develop if there is either

- decreased coronary flow or
- increased demand of more oxygen.

What influences coronary blood flow?

- *Perfusion pressure.* Diastolic pressure determines perfusion pressure in the coronaries. For example, in cases of severe hypotension and shock, the drop in pressure may lead to myocardial ischemia.

    The coronary pressure necessary to secure flow is also influenced by the resistance offered by the myocardium. Coronary flow from the left coronary will be mainly diastolic since the contracted left ventricular myocardium in systole will interrupt the flow because of the level of systolic pressure. The right coronary artery, perfusing the right ventricle, will encounter lower resistance from the low right ventricular pressure, and the flow is both systolic and diastolic.

Right & Left Coronary Flow Patterns

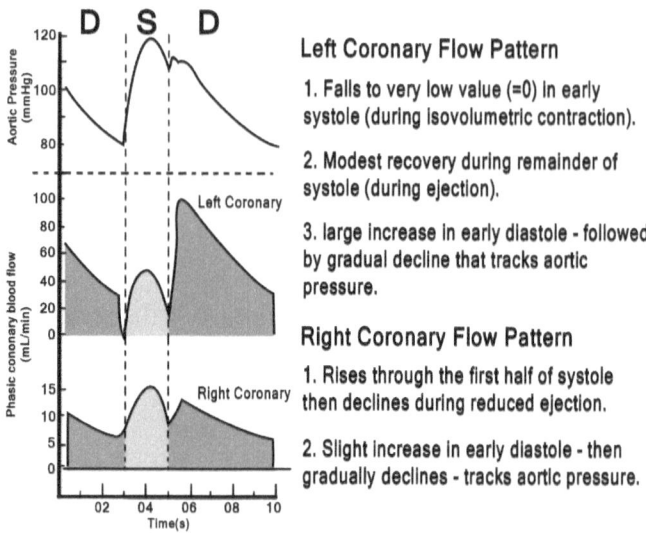

Fig. 10.1. Right and left coronary flow in systole and diastole.

- *Coronary vascular resistance.* Vasoconstriction will decrease flow by narrowing the vessel lumen. The resistance will increase to the fourth power of the change in diameter.
- *Diastolic filling time per minute.* Coronary flow is mainly diastolic (during systole, the contracted myocardium increases coronary resistance and impedes flow). The duration of diastole influences coronary flow. Tachycardia shortens diastolic time and therefore could decrease coronary flow. For example, if a patient increases heart rate from 80 beats per minute to 110, diastolic filling time will decrease by 37%.

In many conditions, either because demand is increased (for example, cardiac hypertrophy) or the ability to increase supply is limited, the myocardium may start operating in an anaerobic manner.

What factors influence and could decrease O_2 supply to the myocardium?

- Inadequate blood O_2 supply
    - *Anemia.* In severe anemia, O_2 saturation may be normal, but the decrease in hemoglobin decreases the amount of O_2 available for transport.
    - *Hypoxia.* Lowering of alveolar pO_2—for example, at high altitude where barometric pressure will be lower—alveolar pO_2 will decrease proportionately resulting in lowering of arterial pO_2. The resulting hypoxia will decrease availability of O_2 for the myocardium.

- Inadequate coronary flow
    - *Coronary spasm.* Coronary vasoconstriction (i.e. Prinzmetal angina) will decrease flow to the fourth power of the change in vessel diameter.
    - Coronary obstruction is caused by an atherosclerotic plaque.

What are the factors that influence O_2 demand by the myocardium?

- *Heart rate.* Myocyte contraction is the primary factor determining myocardial oxygen

consumption. Doubling heart rate will double MVO_2 because ventricular myocytes are generating twice the number of tension cycles per minute.
- ○ *Muscle mass.* The greater size of the muscle mass necessitates an increase in O_2 supply.
- ○ *Contractile force.* Increasing inotropy also increases MVO_2 because the tension development as well as the magnitude of tension are increased.
- ○ *Wall tension.* The LaPlace relationship says that wall tension is proportional to the product of intraventricular pressure and ventricular radius.

From a practical perspective, heart rate and systolic pressure are the most important and easy-to-measure factors that affect myocardial oxygen consumption.

The product of heart rate and systolic arterial pressure, also known as double product, is an indirect measure of myocardial O_2 consumption.

What additional changes take place in the presence of an ischemic myocardium?

What are the pathophysiological alterations during an episode of myocardial ischemia?

- *Subendocardial ischemia.* Coronary vessels traverse the myocardium from epicardium to endocardium and are terminal vessels. It is more likely that ischemia of the subendocardium will begin with increased subendocardial pressure or any decrease in flow.

- *Decreased compliance.* The biochemical substrate that results in the stiffening of the myocardium is not clear but is a common consequence of subendocardial ischemia to alter the pressure-volume relationship of the ventricle. Clinically, these changes result in elevation of ventricular end-diastolic pressure during an episode of angina.

- Hypoxic conditions lead to diminished intracellular concentrations of ATP.

- *Regional alterations in contractility* at peak exercise are easily seen as transient changes in ventricular wall motion.

- *Decrease action potential upstroke (phase 0) velocity.* This leads to decreased conduction velocity that can contribute to arrhythmias.

Ischemia may occur without pain and is referred as **silent ischemia.** Silent ischemia is easily documented with ambulatory ECG monitoring. Some studies have shown that the episodes are short and have a circadian pattern, with most episodes occurring shortly after arousal or waking during the night. It has also been shown that up to 80% of ischemic episodes are silent.

Silent ischemia can be demonstrated with

- asymptomatic ST-segment deviation detected during continuous ambulatory electrocardiographic monitoring,
- stress-provoked asymptomatic electrocardiographic changes during exercise-tolerance test, and

- inducible perfusion defects or reversible regional wall-motion abnormalities during stress-imaging techniques.

Ischemic episodes may develop with or without documentable coronary artery disease. If coronary artery disease is present, the degree of vessel obstruction is usually greater than 60%.

What are the tests commonly used to diagnose myocardial ischemia?

In addition to a careful, detailed history and clinical evaluation, a number of diagnostic tests are commonly used. These tests use the pathophysiological alterations or detectable anatomical changes to make the diagnosis. For example:

- Exercise electrocardiogram determines the existence of ischemia through the abnormalities in repolarization (ST-T) that develop when subendocardial ischemia appears.

- Thallium 201 detects abnormalities in perfusion that are seen in nuclear images during exercise.

- Stress echocardiogram detects regional abnormalities in wall motion that appear when segments of the myocardium become ischemic.

- Radiographic tests identify the amount of calcium deposit in the coronaries as a diagnostic sign.

Each of these tests have their own sensitivity and specificity.

TREATMENT

The main goals of treatment in angina pectoris are to

- decrease myocardial oxygen consumption and
- increase coronary blood supply.

The following approaches are available:

MEDICAL TREATMENT

Drugs can

- ○ Decrease O_2 demand
  Beta-blockers. These drugs decrease myocardial O_2 consumption by causing a lower heart rate and lowering arterial pressure. A large body of evidence demonstrated that beta-blockers reduce the morbidity and mortality (fewer symptoms, less disability, and longer life).
- ○ Decrease O_2 demand by reducing afterload
  - Calcium channel blockers
  - Nitrates
  - ACE inhibitors

All these drugs are commonly used in chronic stable angina.

In addition to the above

- Cholesterol-lowering agents
- Low-dose aspirin
- *Exercise.* Muscle conditioning will lower blood pressure and resting heart rate as well as promote development of coronary artery collaterals.
- Treating risk factors like
  - ○ hypertension,

- ○ smoking cessation, and
- ○ weight control.

THERAPEUTIC INTERVENTIONS

- *Coronary bypass surgery.* Both PCI and CABG are more effective than medical management at relieving symptoms. CABG is superior to PCI for some patients with multivessel disease.

- *Coronary angioplasty.* Patients with anatomically suitable lesions are candidates for percutaneous transluminal coronary angioplasty and coronary stenting to relieve the obstruction. Restenosis is the major complication, with symptomatic restenosis occurring in 20–25% of patients. Restenosis mostly occurs during the first six months after the procedure and can be managed by repeat angioplasty.

    The use of stents and drug-eluting stents can remarkably reduce the rate of in-stent restenosis. With the introduction of these drug-coated stents, patients with multivessel disease can be treated with percutaneous revascularization.

CASE 10 QUESTIONS

1. An episode of angina usually causes

    a. Increased compliance
    b. Decreased compliance
    c. Increased ventricular volume
    d. Decreased LV diastolic pressure

2. During an episode of angina, the action potential of ischemic myocardium will show

    a. Changed slope of phase 1
    b. Decreased slope of phase 4
    c. Decreased upstroke velocity of phase 0
    d. Increased action potential amplitude

3. Traveling to high altitude decreases pO_2 because

    a. Barometric pressure is lower as altitude increases
    b. O_2 concentration in air decreases
    c. Humidity in air increases
    d. pCO_2 in air increases

4. If the radius of the left ventricle increases because ventricular dilatation

    a. Myocardial O_2 demand will decrease
    b. LV wall tension will decrease
    c. LV wall tension will increase
    d. LV contractility will decrease

5. If a patient has a GI bleed and his Hgb drops from 14 gms to 6

    a. pO_2 will decrease
    b. O_2 saturation will decrease

c. Dissolved O_2 will increase
   d. Total O_2 content delivered will decrease

6. Increased left ventricular afterload is likely to

   a. Cause coronary vasodilatation
   b. Alter transmyocardial pressure
   c. Lower end-diastolic pressure
   d. Decrease ventricular work

CASE NO. 11: ACUTE MYOCARDIAL INFARCTION

Mr. RB is a sixty-year-old male that, on a Monday morning, on his way to work, begins to notice mild epigastric discomfort accompanied by nausea. When he reaches the office, he now feels that the problem is anterior and epigastric pain that radiates to his left shoulder. Few minutes later, the pain intensifies; he remains nauseated and vomits once. His coworkers note that he is pale and perspiring profusely.

Further information indicated that in the past, he was being treated for elevated cholesterol and mildly elevated blood pressure.

They immediately called 911, and in twelve minutes, he is being transported to the emergency department of a local hospital. An ECG had been transmitted by the paramedics, and it shows an acute inferior myocardial infarction.

His family history is significant in that his father died of an acute MI at age sixty-six and a brother has elevated cholesterol and recent unstable angina leading to a quadruple coronary bypass. A sister has elevated cholesterol.

Upon arrival to the ED, his pulse rate is 33 per minute, his blood pressure 90/60, and respiration 28 per minute.

He is in acute distress now with severe chest pain.

- Examination of head and neck is unremarkable.
- Arterial pulses are weak.
- Auscultation of lungs is unremarkable.
- Cardiovascular examination reveals soft heart sounds and no murmurs or rubs.
- Abdomen is soft and bowel sounds are normal.

A new ECG is taken upon arrival to the ED, suggesting that the patient is having an acute coronary event demonstrating an acute injury current with ST segment elevation in leads 2, 3, AVF, and ST depression V1–V3, indicating an inferoposterior injury most likely resulting from a right coronary occlusion

Pulse oximetry reveals a saturation of 92%. He is immediately give two milligrams of morphine sulfate and one milligram of atropine sulfate intravenously, and nasal O_2 is given. Blood is drawn to measure the various biomarkers. But the presentation is typical and the ECG diagnostic that treatment measures are implemented.

In acute myocardial infarction, time is of the essence to save the ischemic myocardium. He is transported to the cardiac catheterization laboratory where angiogram is done and an infusion of TPA is started.

The patient is subsequently admitted to the coronary care unit, where he recovered uneventfully.

DISCUSSION

The case under discussion represents the classic presentation of an acute myocardial infarction.

Coronary disease will manifest itself in different manners, often as the following:

- Silent ischemia, discussed earlier
- Angina pectoris, discussed earlier—results from the narrowing of a coronary vessel that disturbs the balance between myocardial O_2 needs and O_2 supply

- Acute coronary syndromes (ACS)
    º Unstable angina
    º Acute myocardial infarction

A basic review of the development and progression of coronary artery disease is presented here.

Obstructive coronary lesions may eventually progress and cause myocardial tissue death. This is a long process, and studies have demonstrated that individuals can show evidence of cholesterol deposits and early plaque formation in late teens.

The pathophysiology of this progression can be briefly described as follows:

The first step in the development and progression of coronary disease is the formation of the atherosclerotic plaque. This involves five different steps:

- Accumulation of low-density lipoprotein (LDL) in the intima
- Recruitment of monocytes and macrophages in the developing plaque
- Uptake of oxidized LDL by macrophage scavenger receptors
- Transformation of macrophages into foam cells
- Formation of a fibrous cap containing smooth muscle cells, which permits stabilization of the plaque

DEVELOPMENT OF AN ACUTE CORONARY SYNDROME

Progression of coronary disease to the development of an acute coronary syndrome necessitates plaque erosion or plaque rupture that facilitates thrombus formation.

Plaque rupture occurs where the cap is thinnest and most infiltrated by foam cells (macrophages). Only extremely thin fibrous caps are at risk of rupturing, and they are less calcified than plaques responsible for stable angina. They are often referred as culprit lesions.

Once the plaque ruptures, the stage is set for localized thrombosis to develop. Local factors influencing the growth of a thrombus include the following:

- A rough plaque surface that stimulates the development of an occlusive thrombus.
- More platelet deposition and thrombus formation occur.
- Vasospasm.
- Various systemic factors such as levels of epinephrine, serum cholesterol, and impaired fibrinolysis influence the formation of the thrombus.
- Localized and unresolved myocardial ischemia will lead to necrosis and an acute myocardial infarction.

As a result, the following events will then happen:

- After ischemia occurs, the myocardium switches immediately from aerobic glycolysis to anaerobic glycolysis, resulting in the reduced ability to produce high-energy phosphates such as ATP and creatinine phosphate.

- At this point, the lack of the energy and lactate accumulation result in cessation of contraction within sixty seconds of ischemia (i.e. vessel occlusion).

Two types of infarction may occur:

Acute myocardial infarction *(ST elevation MI)* refers to regional myocardial necrosis, secondary to occlusion of an epicardial artery.

Acute myocardial infarction (subendocardial) is referred as ST depression. MI will be discussed in a separate case.

Myocardial infarction causes migration of macrophages and monocytes.

Changes in hemodynamics are determined primarily by the magnitude of myocyte loss, the stimulation of the sympathetic nervous system and renin-angiotensin-aldosterone system, and the release of natriuretic peptides.

The area where the infarct occurs is associated with the area of the distribution of the occluded vessel. The area of distribution varies considerably.

- Left main coronary artery occlusion generally results in a large anterolateral infarct.

- Left anterior descending artery occlusion causes an infarction of the anterior wall. There is often extension to the anterior portion of the ventricular septum.

- Right coronary occlusion will commonly cause an infarction of the inferior wall of the left ventricle. If the RCA dominates, its posterior branch will cause involvement of the posterior wall.

PATHOPHYSIOLOGICAL EVENTS AFTER THE ONSET OF A MYOCARDIAL INFARCTION

Shortly after the onset of myocardial death, the following will happen:

- *Stunned myocardium.* This affects some section of the myocardium corresponding to the area of distribution of the affected vessel. This is a contractile abnormality that may persist for about two weeks, even after ischemia has been relieved and reperfusion achieved. The mechanism is as follows :
    - Immediately after total ischemia occurs, the myocardium switches from aerobic glycolysis to anaerobic glycolysis.
    - This reduces the ability to produce ATP and creatinine phosphate.
    - The lack of the energy and lactate accumulation results in cessation of contraction.
    - Subsequent to the period of myocardial stunning, and in approximately thirty minutes, after the onset of total ischemia, the damage becomes irreversible.

- *Postinfarction left ventricular remodeling.* After thirty minutes to one hour, the irreversible and localized myocardial damage will result in a number of pathophysiological changes.

The acute loss of myocardium induces a unique pattern of remodeling involving both the infarcted border zone and remote noninfarcted myocardium.

Postinfarction remodeling has been divided into

- *Early phase (within seventy-two hours).* The early phase involves expansion of the infarct zone, which may result in early ventricular rupture or aneurysm formation. Infarct expansion results from the degradation of the intermyocyte collagen struts by serine proteases and the activation of matrix metalloproteinases (MMPs) released from neutrophils.

Infarct expansion occurs within hours of myocyte injury and results in wall thinning and ventricular dilatation, which causes the elevation of diastolic and systolic wall stress.

The resulting wall stress is a major determinant of ventricular performance.

Preservation of cardiac output and stroke volume generates a number of responses by the noninfarcted remote myocardium:

- Infarct expansion causes the deformation of the border zone and remote myocardium and augments shortening.
- The sympathetic adrenergic system is stimulated and increases catecholamine production.
- The renin-angiotensin-aldosterone system is activated, stimulating the production of atrial and brain natriuretic peptides (ANP and BNP).
- Augmented shortening and increased heart rate from sympathetic stimulation result in hyperkinesis of the noninfarcted myocardium.
- In addition, the natriuretic peptides reduce intravascular volume and systemic vascular resistance, normalize ventricular filling, and improve pump function.

- *Late phase (beyond seventy-two hours).* Late remodeling involves the left ventricle globally and is associated with dilatation, distortion of ventricular shape, and hypertrophy.

Ventricular remodeling may continue for weeks or months until the distending forces are counterbalanced by the tensile strength of the collagen scar. This balance affecting remodeling is determined by the

- size, location, transmural penetration of the tissue loss;
- the extent of myocardial stunning; and
- the patency of the infarct-related artery.

Failure to normalize increased wall stresses results in progressive dilatation and further deterioration in contractile function.

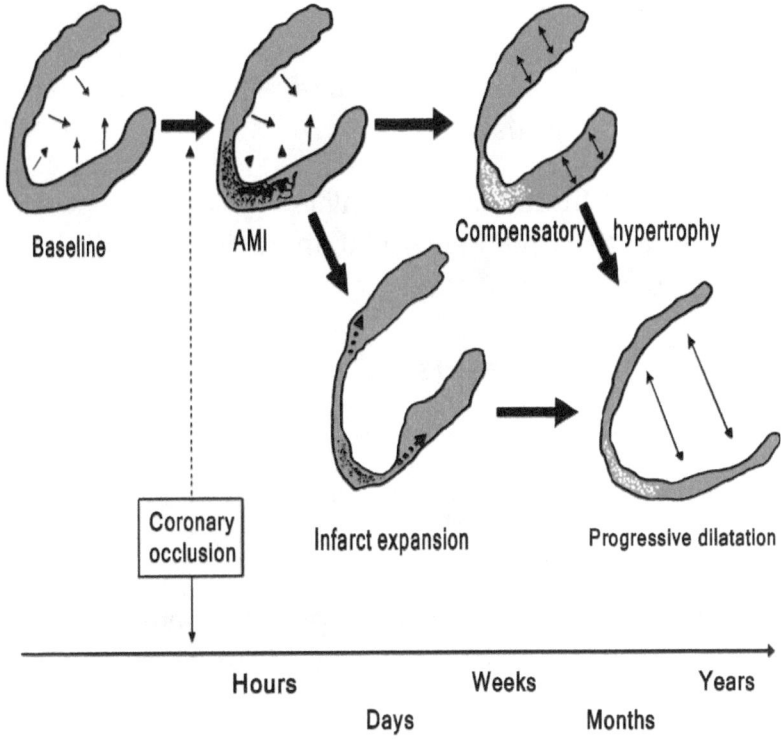

Fig. 11.3

In addition to the hemodynamic changes mentioned, the ischemic myocardium may create electrical instability and anatomical changes that may lead to interruption of the normal conduction pathways and a number of other complications. They will be discussed in subsequent cases.

The ST segment elevation representing epicardial injury will resolve over time and serves as an index of reperfusion.

- Complete resolution of ST elevation is accompanied by thirty-day mortality of 2.9%.
- Partial resolution has a thirty-day mortality of 5.8% and

- No ST resolution has a thirty-day mortality of 10.2% and 11% six-month mortality.

The prognosis for acute myocardial infarction can be summarized as follows:

- Newer treatment modalities have substantially decreased the in-hospital mortality as well as the hospital length of stay.

- About 50% of the deaths occur prior to arrival at the hospital.

- An additional 5–10% of survivors die within the first year after their myocardial infarction.

- Approximately half of all patients with an MI are rehospitalized within one year of their event.

- Overall, prognosis is highly variable and depends largely on the extent of the infarct, the residual left ventricular function, and whether the patient underwent revascularization.

  Better prognosis is associated with the following factors:

- Successful early reperfusion (ST elevation MI [STEMI] goals—patient arrival to fibrinolysis infusion within thirty minutes *or* patient arrival to percutaneous coronary intervention [PCI] within ninety minutes)
- Preserved left ventricular function
- Short-term and long-term treatment with beta-blockers, aspirin, and angiotensin-converting enzyme (ACE) inhibitors

Poorer prognosis is associated with the following factors:

- Advanced age (Age older than sixty-five years is associated with higher mortality.)
- Diabetes mellitus
- Previous vascular disease (i.e., cerebrovascular disease or peripheral vascular disease)
- Risk factors for cardiac disease, previous coronary disease (i.e., smoking, obesity)
- ST segment deviation ≥ 0.5 mm,
- ≥ 2 episodes of angina in the last twenty-four hours,
- Delayed or unsuccessful reperfusion
- Poorly preserved left ventricular function (the strongest predictor of outcome)
- Evidence of congestive heart failure
- Elevated B-type natriuretic peptide (BNP) levels
- Elevated high-sensitive C-reactive protein (hs-CRP), a nonspecific inflammatory marker
- Depression
- Magnitude of ST elevation and reciprocal changes
- Duration of ST elevation
- Time for the regression of ST elevation after thrombolytic therapy
- Ejection fraction
- Troponin levels
- CK-MB levels
- Number of Q waves (extent of infarction)
- Extent of wall motion abnormalities

Biomarkers

Biomarkers are critical in the diagnosis of a myocardial infarction. Their elevation is indicative of myocardial necrosis, and the magnitude of the elevation serve as a general indicator of the magnitude of tissue loss. The enclosed table shows when they rise and peak and how many days they remain elevated.

MARKERS	INCREASE	PEAK LEVEL	PERSISTANCE
TROPONIN	2-6 hr	48 hr	4-14 days
CK-MB	4-6 hr	24 hr	2-3 days
MYOGLOBIN	1 hr	2-12 hr	24-36 hr
LDH1	12-16 hr	48-72 hr	10 days

Table 11.1

Cardiac troponins control the calcium-mediated interaction of actin and myosin. It exists in three isoforms: troponin C, troponin I, and troponin T. Troponin C exists in all muscle tissues. However, cTnI is completely specific for the heart. Elevation of troponin has a sensitivity of 33% from 0–2 hours, 50% from 2–4 hours, 75% from 4–8 hours, and approaching 100% from 8 hours after onset of chest pain. Elevated troponin is an independent predictor of mortality.

CK-MB levels become elevated in 4 to 6 hours, peak at 10 to 24 hours, and return to normal within 3 to 4 days after an acute myocardial infarction. They are not as predictive as troponin. In the presence of skeletal muscle injury, specificity is low and has low sensitivity in the first 6 hours after onset of symptoms.

Myoglobin is found in skeletal and cardiac muscle. Myoglobin typically rises 2–4 hours after onset of infarction, peaks at 6–12 hours, and returns to normal within 24–36 hours. It lacks specificity. Myoglobin has only achieved 90% sensitivity for acute MI, so the negative predictive value of myoglobin is not high.

Complications following an MI can be either mechanical or electrical and will be discussed in following cases.

Electrical complications. About 90% of patients who have an acute myocardial infarction develop some form of cardiac arrhythmia during or immediately after the event. In 25% of patients, such rhythm abnormalities manifest within the first twenty-four hours. The risk of serious arrhythmias, such as ventricular fibrillation, is greatest in the first hour and declines thereafter. The incidence of arrhythmia is higher with an ST elevation myocardial infarction (STEMI) and lower with a non–ST elevation myocardial infarction (NSTEMI).

Mechanical complications. The following table illustrates the frequency of some of the major mechanical complications.

	FREE WALL RUPTURE	VENTRICULAR SEPTAL DEFECT	PAPILLARY MUSCLE RUPT	R.V. INFARCTION
WITHOUT REPERFUSION	1 – 6 %	1 – 3 %	+/- 1 %	> 15 % to 40 %
WITH REPERFUSION	1 – 3 %	0.2 %		

Table 11.2

In cases that follow, we will present examples and offer a more detailed discussion of some of the complications.

TREATMENT

The following is a brief review of accepted treatment modalities for patients with an acute myocardial infarction:

- **Management of pain and anxiety**

    Morphine is one of the best drugs for this purpose. It relieves pain and anxiety. In addition, it has some hemodynamic effect such as some decrease in preload and some inotropic properties

- **Restoration of flow**

    As discussed previously, myocardial death occurs rapidly if coronary flow cease. Plaque rupture leads to clot formation in the involved area. Efforts to restore flow must take place in very few hours from the onset of symptoms. Time is inversely proportional to mortality as shown in this table

Time Delay	Mortality
<60 min	1%
60–75 min	3.7%
76–90min	4.7%
> 90min	6.4%
not done	14.1%

Table 11.3

Reperfusion can be achieved through the following:

- *Mechanically.* Coronary angioplasty is the preferred mechanical method to achieve reperfusion and with the insertion of a stent to establish long-term perfusion through the affected vessel.
- *Pharmacological.* Intravenous administration of drugs such as tPA. Fibrinolytic (thrombolytic) therapy is capable of reestablishing antegrade blood flow in nearly 75% of patients when administered within the first two hours of symptom onset.

Currently, coronary angioplasty is favored over thrombolytic therapy. Multiple circumstances, however, may influence the choice, such as availability of experienced operators and other logistical issues. In older individuals, coronary angioplasty is preferred because of the increased risks of intracranial hemorrhage caused by thrombolytic therapy.

- **Anticoagulant therapy**

    Since clot formation develops in the site of the plaque rupture, sustained therapeutic levels of anticoagulation are essential to prevent the recurrence of clot formation.

    Heparin. The recommended dose is an intravenous (IV) bolus of 60 U/kg and infusion adjusted to maintain the activated partial thromboplastin time (aPTT) at 1.5–2 times the control value.

    Low molecular weight heparin. This is an alternative to heparin. In patients younger than seventy-five years, the recommendation is a 30-mg IV bolus followed by 1 mg/kg subcutaneously every 12 hours. For those over seventy-five years, the dose is 0.75 mg/kg every 12 hours, and no bolus is administered.

- **Reduction of platelet aggregation**

    Increased platelet aggregation at the site of the plaque rupture and the thrombus formation have a direct impact on the outcomes of fibrinolytic therapy.

    Fibrinolytic agents given in conjunction with antithrombin and antiplatelet agents help maintain vessel patency once the clot has been dissolved. The following are commonly used:

- ▶ *Aspirin.* It inhibits platelet aggregation. The recommended dose is 162–325 mg of chewable aspirin.
- ▶ *Clopidogrel.* Also inhibits platelets. There is evidence for benefit of adding clopidogrel to aspirin in patients undergoing fibrinolytic therapy.

- **Reduction of afterload**

    Afterload plays an important role in influencing myocardial work and myocardial oxygen consumption and, as a result, improves prognosis.

    Systemic vasodilators decrease left ventricular systolic wall tension (ventricular afterload) by reducing aortic impedance and/or by reducing cardiac venous return. Thus, vasodilators increase cardiac output (CO) by diminishing peripheral vascular resistance (PVR) and/or decrease increased left ventricular end-diastolic pressure (LVEDP) (ventricular preload) by diminishing venous tone. There is also a reduction of myocardial oxygen demand, thereby limiting infarct size and ischemia. The vasodilators produce disparate modifications of cardiac function depending upon their differing alterations of preload versus impedance.

- ***Management of cardiac arrhythmia***

    A number of antiarrhythmic agents are available depending on the type of arrhythmia.

- **_Management of hemodynamic consequences_**

Hypotension and cardiogenic shock are serious complications to be discussed in a subsequent case. Vasopressors are the favored drugs, and in severe cases, use of an intra-aortic balloon becomes indicated (see a following case).

CASE 11 QUESTIONS

1. An MI can result in

   a. Increased end-systolic volume
   b. Decreased cardiac work
   c. Lower peripheral vascular resistance
   d. Increased end-diastolic volume

2. Ventricular remodeling can

   a. Only be caused by coronary disease
   b. Decrease myocardial O_2 consumption
   c. Decrease wall stress
   d. Increase wall stress

3. Plaque rupture is often associated with

   a. Thick plaques
   b. Calcified plaques
   c. Mild coronary artery narrowing
   d. Macrophage presence

4. Prognosis of an acute MI is often influenced by

   a. ST segment deviation ≥ 0.5 mm,
   b. Normal enzyme level
   c. Successful revascularization
   d. Elevated BNP level

5. The following regarding an acute myocardial infarction is correct:

   a. Around 10% of the deaths occur prior to arrival at the hospital
   b. One year mortality is 10%

c. Around 50% of survivors will be readmitted to the hospital within one year
d. Ventricular function is not a factor in one-year survival

CASE NO. 12: VENTRICULAR ANEURYSM

A sixty-four-year-old male who had suffered a large myocardial infarction sixteen months ago presents to the office stating that in the last three months, he has noticed a marked decrease in exercise tolerance. It has become progressively worse in the last few weeks and is starting to limit his activities of daily living. He easily becomes short of breath and has noted some shortness of breath when in bed.

Physical examination reveals the following:

BP = 140/90, P = 94 per minute.

Apical impulse is very diffused; an S3 and S4 are heard at the apex.

The ECG demonstrated an extensive anterior MI, and the ST segment shows elevation in precordial leads.

The patient underwent an ECG treadmill test that showed an increase in the ST segment elevation or the development of elevation. The increase in heart rate and contractility affect the myocardium and create transient ischemia.

DISCUSSION

Ventricular aneurysm is one of the many complications that may occur after a myocardial infarction. They usually arise from a weakened tissue in a ventricular wall that stretches as a result of the repetitive systolic pressure applied to the endocardial layers. The changes in ventricular geometry alter cardiac function and can lead to congestive heart failure.

The aneurysm is usually nonrupturing because it has abundant scar tissue. This is opposed to pseudoaneurysm that reflect a myocardial hematoma and a partial rupture at risk of additional rupture.

The persistent ST elevation seen often in patients with ventricular aneurysm results from the tension that each systole places in the healthy myocardium at the junction with the scar tissue. The persistence of ST elevation months after an MI or its marked increase during exercise is strongly suggestive of a ventricular aneurysm or a significant area of dyskinesia or akinesia.

The cause of a ventricular aneurysm is most often a myocardial infarction, although other factors may lead to its deveopment—for example, cardiomyopathies, such as Chagas disease, which causes a large area of scar tissue that results in the formation of an anuerysm.

PATHOPHYSIOLOGICAL CHANGES IN VENTRICULAR ANEURYSM

The pathophysiology associated with a ventricular aneurysm is the consequence of the altered morphology and geometry of the left ventricle. The following changes can be observed:

- Increased left ventricular end-diastolic volume.
- Increased transmural pressure and mean systolic force.
- Isometric rate of pressure rise is uniformly decreased.
- Fiber shortening velocity and distance are moderately depressed.
- Stroke output and cardiac output are often reduced.
- Cardiac contractility exhibits either paradoxical systolic expansion or apparent lack of motion (akinesia) or both.
- The degree of shortening distance required of the myofiber to maintain stroke volume exceeds

physiological limits, and cardiac enlargement (Starling mechanism) must ensue to maintain adequate ejection of blood.

In addition to the hemodynamic changes that often lead to congestive heart failure, the risk of embolization is seriously increased. The development of large areas of akinetic myocardium promotes blood stasis and formation of clot that may dislodge and embolize in the arterial system.

Another potential complication is the development of ventricular arrhythmias as a result of the electrical instability created by the stretching of healthy myocardium in the area surrounding scar tissue.

TREATMENT

Treatment should include prevention of embolization through anticoagulation, management of heart failure, and potential cardiac surgery to resect the area of scar tissue and improve cardiac function.

CASE 12 QUESTIONS

1. The presence of a ventricular aneurysm will

    a. Decrease peripheral vascular resistance
    b. Decrease preload
    c. Increase end-systolic volume
    d. Increase end-diastolic volume

2. The tissue in the area of the ventricular aneurysm is likely to be

    a. Hyperkinetic
    b. Normokinetic
    c. Akinetic

3. In a patient with a large aneurysm

    a. Fiber shortening velocity is normal
    b. Fiber shortening in normal myocardium will be depressed
    c. In the area of the aneurysm, fiber shortening will be depressed
    d. Stroke volume will be increased

4. In a patient with a large ventricular arneurysm, the following arrhythmia can frequently ocurr

    a. Atrial flutter
    b. Atrial fibrillation
    c. Ventricular tachycardia
    d. Heart block

5. Of the following myocardial diseases, which one is more likely to develop an aneurysm?

    a. Rheumatic fever
    b. Coksakie
    c. Chagas
    d. HIV

6. The big difference between ventricular aneurysm and pseudoaneurysm is

    a. Size
    b. Location
    c. Cause
    d. Rupture

CASE NO. 13: UNSTABLE ANGINA

Mr. JT is a sixty-five-year-old retired high school teacher with a history of obesity, moderate essential hypertension, and occasional episodes of exercise-induced angina. On a Sunday afternoon and while playing golf, he develops an episode of angina while sitting in the golf cart. The pain is relieved by a nitroglycerin tablet. He decides to terminate the game and drives home.

That evening, while resting in bed, he again develops chest pain, but this time, it is not completely relieved by nitroglycerin. His wife transports him to a local hospital, where an ECG is taken that demonstrates ST segment depression on leads 1, AVL and V4 to V6 while the patient reports chest pain.

He reports that in recent weeks, he has noted an increase in the number of episodes of angina while walking, and one night, he developed chest pain while in bed, relieved by nitroglycerin tablet.

The diagnosis of unstable angina is made, and he is transferred to a local tertiary care hospital, where he is scheduled for a cardiac catheterization that afternoon. Evaluation of the angiogram demonstrates the need for multiple coronary bypasses, and surgery is performed the following morning.

DISCUSSION

This patient demonstrates many of the classical features of unstable angina:

- ○ Accelerating frequency of angina episodes
- ○ Angina appearing at rest
- ○ Nocturnal episodes of angina

Unstable angina belongs to the spectrum of acute coronary syndromes (ACSs), in which there is no detectable release of the biomarkers that indicate myocardial necrosis. It should be approached as a medical emergency since the risk of myocardial infarction is elevated.

PATHOGENESIS OF ACUTE CORONARY SYNDROMES

The combination of a ruptured atherosclerotic plaque with a superimposed thrombi is present in many cases of unstable angina. There are major differences between stable and unstable angina, and so is the pathophysiology.

- In *stable angina*, the fundamental pathophysiology is fixed coronary stenosis that compromises blood flow. The pain develops when myocardial oxygen demand increases above available O_2 supply. The myocardium becomes ischemic, but the need of additional O_2 decreases when demand decreases.
- In *unstable angina*, other factors appear and play major roles. Such factors include the following:
    - Supply-demand mismatch
    - Plaque disruption or rupture
    - Thrombosis
    - Vasoconstriction
    - Cyclical flow

SUPPLY-DEMAND MISMATCH

Excess oxygen demand from increased myocardial workload or wall stress is responsible for nearly all cases of stable angina and perhaps one-third of all episodes of unstable angina.

PLAQUE DISRUPTION

The following events take place:

- Accumulation of macrophages and foam cells, within atherosclerotic plaques. The LDL-C in foam cells is cytotoxic, procoagulant, and chemotactic.
- As the atherosclerotic plaque grows, production of macrophage proteases and neutrophil elastases within the plaque can cause thinning of the fibromuscular cap that covers the lipid core.
- Increasing plaque instability, blood-flow shear, and circumferential wall stress lead to plaque rupture, especially at the junction of the cap and the vessel wall.
- Moderate to large plaque disruptions commonly result in unstable angina or acute infarction.

VASOCONSTRICTION and THROMBOSIS

Most patients with acute coronary syndrome have recurrent transient reduction in coronary blood supply because of vasoconstriction and thrombus formation at the site of atherosclerotic plaque rupture.

Platelets then aggregate in response to exposed vessel wall collagen or local aggregates (e.g., thromboxane and adenosine diphosphate). Platelets also release substances that promote vasoconstriction and production of thrombin. In a reciprocating fashion, thrombin is a potent agonist for further platelet activation, and it stabilizes thrombi by converting fibrinogen to fibrin.

ACS may involve a clot in flux enlarging, breaking off, and embolizing. The nonocclusive thrombus of unstable angina can become transiently or persistently occlusive. Depending on the duration of the occlusion, the presence of collateral vessels and the area of myocardium perfused, recurrent unstable angina, non–Q wave MI (NQMI), or Q-wave MI can result.

TREATMENT

Initial medical treatment attempts the following:

1. **Decrease O_2 consumption**

    - Beta-adrenergic blocking agents
    - Nitrates

2. **Decrease platelet aggregation**

    - Aspirin
    - PSY12 inhibitors (thienopyridines [clopidogrel, prasugrel], nonthienopyridines [ticagrelor])
    - GP IIb/IIIa antagonists

3. **Anticoagulation**

    - Heparin
    - Direct thrombin inhibitors

4. **Interventional treatment**

    - Angiogram and angioplasty
    - Stent insertion
    - Coronary bypass surgery

CASE 13 QUESTIONS

1. Plaque rupture usually occurs in

    a. Thick calcified plaques
    b. Thinnest portion of
    c. Big plaques
    d. Small-vessel plaques

2. Factors involved in the pathophysiology of unstable angina include the following:

    a. Supply-demand mismatch
    b. Plaque rupture
    c. Thrombosis
    d. Hemolysis
    e. a, b, c

3. Production of macrophage proteases cause thinning of the fibromuscular cap that covers the lipid core.

    a. True
    b. False

4. Depending on the duration of the occlusion, the presence of collateral vessels, and the area of myocardium perfused, the following could happen:

    a. Recurrent unstable angina
    b. Restoration of normal flow
    c. Q-wave MI can result
    d. Atrial fibrillation will develop

5. Unstable angina

    a. Will always have new Q waves in the ECG
    b. Biomarkers will always be abnormal
    c. ST segment and T wave abnormalities will be observed
    d. Arrhythmia will always be observed

6. Coronary vasoconstriction

    a. Is common
    b. Is rare
    c. A minor feature of unstable angina
    d. Often before thrombus formation

CASE NO. 14: ACUTE MI AND HEART BLOCK

Mr. RG is a busy seventy-two-year-old real estate agent who wakes up one morning and is on his way to work when he begins to notice mild epigastric discomfort accompanied by nausea. When he reaches the office, he now feels anterior and epigastric pain that radiates to his left shoulder. Few minutes later, the pain intensifies; he remains nauseated and vomits once. His coworkers note that he is pale and perspiring profusely. They immediately called 911, and in twelve minutes, he is being transported to the emergency department of a local hospital.

An ECG had been transmitted by the paramedics, and it shows an acute inferior myocardial infarction.

Upon arrival to the ED, his pulse rate is 33 per minute, his blood pressure is 90/60, and respiration is 28 per minute.

He is in acute distress, now with severe chest pain.

- Examination of head and neck is unremarkable.
- Arterial pulses are weak.
- Auscultation of lungs is unremarkable.
- Cardiovascular examination reveals soft heart sounds and no rubs or murmurs.

A repeat ECG is shown below.

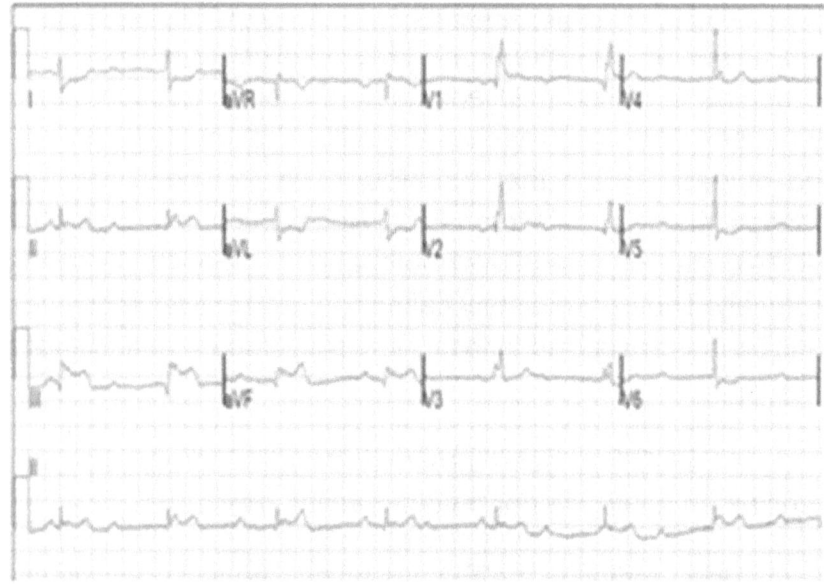

Fig 14 -1 A repeat ECG shows P waves at a rate of 70 per minute and QRS at a rate of 40 per minute, with right bundle branch block and Q waves in and AVF of 40 msec, accompanied by injury current in 2, 3, and AVF, indicating an acute inferior myocardial infarction. There is no temporal correlation between P and QRS, indicating complete AV block

The patient is given one milligram of atropine IV and returns to 1:1 conduction. He is transferred to the catheterization laboratory, where he undergoes a successful angioplasty of the RCA and placement of one stent. His recovery was uneventful and was discharged in five days. His heart block never returned, but his right bundle branch block remained unchanged.

DISCUSSION

This case exemplifies complete heart block in the setting of an acute myocardial infarction and will be discussed together.

Complete AV block, occurring in the setting of an acute MI, is a rare complication, and its outcome is determined by the location of the MI and the underlying coronary circulation.

To clarify the topic, a brief review of the coronary circulation to the conduction system of the heart is presented:

- The sinoatrial node is supplied in 73% of cases by the right coronary artery, by the left coronary in 3%, and by both in 23%.

- The atrioventricular node is supplied by the right coronary artery (80% of cases), by the left (10%), and in 10% by both coronary arteries.

- The common bundle is supplied by the left coronary in 73%, by the right coronary artery in 10% of cases by the left, and both coronary arteries in 17%.

- The arteries supplying the right bundle and left bundle are derived from the left coronary artery.

The following are helpful concepts:

- An acute MI that presents with ST elevation in 2, 3, and AVF (as shown in case no. 14) commonly reflects an infarct in the inferior wall of the left ventricle, supplied in most cases by the right coronary artery (RCA) (see above).

- An acute MI with Q waves and ST elevation in the anterior wall, accompanied by bundle branch block(as shown in case no. 15), more commonly represents a left coronary lesion, often the left anterior descending artery.

- Another helpful concept is the duration of the QRS complex in the dominating rhythm, since it helps in understanding prognostic and treatment implications.

- If the QRS complex has a normal duration, it suggests that ventricular depolarization originates in the AV nodal region, and the block is, most likely, in the right coronary.

  A rhythm originating in the AV nodal region

  - Usually has a ventricular rate of 40–50 beats per minute, often able to maintain an adequate cardiac output.
  - Administration of atropine will shorten AV node refractory period and often allows restoration of normal conduction.
  - Atropine will likely accelerate the nodal rhythm.
  - The prognosis is good since the block is usually transient.

- If the QRS is 0.12 seconds in duration or wider, it suggests the following:
  - The rhythm originates in the ventricle (idioventricular rhythm).
  - It requires immediate implantation of a temporary pacemaker.
  - Because of the extent of infarction, it has a poor prognosis.

These concepts help in estimating the location of the coronary occlusion in the presence of a complete heart block in a patient with an acute myocardial infarction.

How often do conduction defects appear in the context of a coronary occlusion, and what is the mortality?

This is shown in the enclosed table.

A bundle branch block appearing during an acute MI is commonly associated with a higher mortality as shown below.

BLOCK	INCIDENCE %	MORTALITY %
RBBB-LEFT ANT.BLOCK	3	31
LBBB	3.3	38.1
RBBB	1.5	21.4
RBBB AND POST.HEMIBLK	2	40
ANY BLOCK	7.3	32.4
COMPLETE A-V BLOCK	4.3	45.2
MOBITZ 1	1.8	11.8
MOBITZ 2	0.3	33.3

Table 14.1

From this data, one could conclude that

- heart block in the setting of an acute anterior infarction has a poor prognosis, usually determined by the size of the infarction and the instability of the supporting rhythm, and

- heart block in the setting of an inferior MI usually has a good prognosis because the supporting rhythm has a faster rate and the block is usually transient.

The hemodynamic consequences of an acute myocardial infarction with heart block are the combination of the physiological damage caused by the infarction and the effect of the bradyarrhythmia resulting from the heart block.

The hemodynamic changes will be the interplay of the

- acute MI that impairs regional contractility, lowers cardiac output, decrease stroke volume, and causes an increase in peripheral vascular resistance, and

- the bradyarrhythmia of heart block, which necessitates increased contractility in order to maintain an adequate cardiac output.

Another helpful concept is the duration of the QRS complex in the dominating rhythm since it helps in understanding prognostic and treatment implications.

- If the QRS complex has a normal duration, it suggests that ventricular depolarization originates in the AV nodal region and the block is, most likely, in the right coronary.

    A rhythm originating in the AV nodal region

    - Usually has a ventricular rate of 40–50 beats per minute, often able to maintain an adequate cardiac output.
    - Administration of atropine will shorten AV node refractory period and often allows restoration of normal conduction.
    - Atropine will likely accelerate the nodal rhythm.
    - The prognosis is good since the block is usually transient.
- If the QRS is 0.12 seconds in duration or wider, it suggests that

- ○ the rhythm originates in the ventricle (idioventricular rhythm),
- ○ it requires immediate implantation of a temporary pacemaker, and
- ○ because of the extent of infarction, it has a poor prognosis.

TREATMENT

- Complete AV block in the setting of an acute inferior infarction is often reversible with IV atropine, and the use of a temporary pacemaker is a good backup system.

- Complete AV block in the setting of an acute anterior MI requires a temporary pacemaker because of the instability of the supporting rhythm and the common unstable hemodynamics of the infarct. If the patient recovers, it is often necessary to implant a permanent pacemaker.

CASE 14 QUESTIONS

1. The AV node is more frequently perfused by

   a. Left coronary artery
   b. Left anterior descending artery
   c. Right coronary artery
   d. Left circumflex artery

2. The bundle branches are more frequently perfused by

   a. Left coronary artery
   b. Left anterior descending artery
   c. Right coronary artery
   d. Left circumflex artery

3. In a patient with complete heart block, the QRS duration is 0.08, suggesting that

   a. The block is in the atrial conduction system
   b. The AV node
   c. The bundle branches
   d. The Purkinje system

4. Reversal to normal conduction after two milligrams of atropine suggests that

   a. The block is in atrial conduction system
   b. The AV node
   c. The bundle branches
   d. The Purkinje system

5. In a patient with an acute anterior MI who develops complete heart block, the following is correct

    a. Prognosis is good after injection of atropine
    b. Prognosis is poor because of the size of the existing hemodynamic compromise
    c. Pacemaker therapy is not necessary
    d. Wenckebach phenomena will be seen in the ECG

6. If a bundle branch block develops in the setting of an acute MI

    a. Atropine therapy will correct the problem
    b. The prognosis is excellent
    c. The mortality is higher than in non-STEMI
    d. Lower than in STEMI

CASE NO. 15: ACUTE MI HYPOTENSION-CARDIOGENIC SHOCK

DD was a seventy-eight-year-old male, a retired college professor, who had been in relatively good health, quite active, and capable of walking two miles a day at a good pace despite his chronic angina that was well under control.

One afternoon, he developed severe acute chest pain that radiated from the precordium to the neck and left arm. He felt dizzy and perspired profusely. His wife promptly called 911 and was transported to a local emergency room and admitted to the ICU.

On admission, his heart rate was 105 beats per minute and his blood pressure 70/50.

He was pale and clammy. Cardiac examination revealed no murmurs and a soft S4. Lungs auscultation showed few basilar rales.

The ECG is shown below:

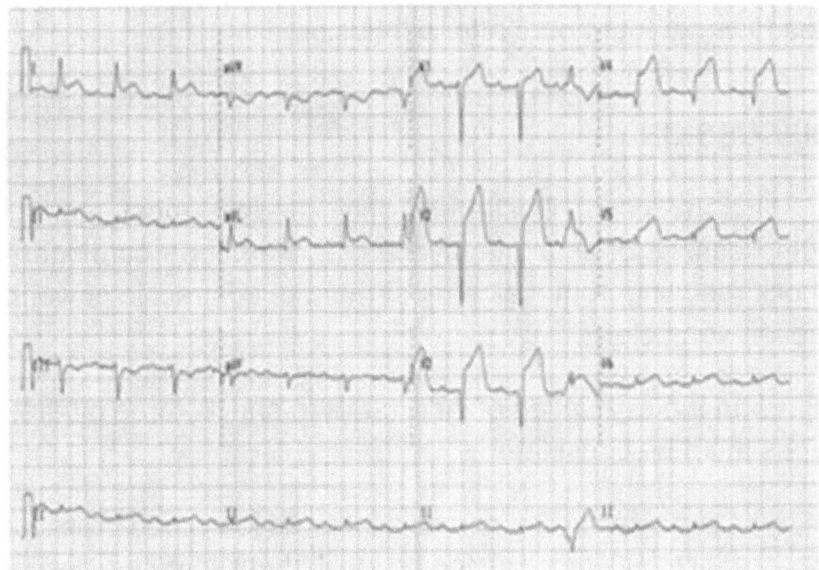

Fig. 16.1. The ECG shows normal sinus rhythm, QS complexes V1 and V2, and an acute injury current in 1, AVL, V1 to V3 with reciprocal changes in 2 and AVF.

The clinical diagnosis was an acute anterior myocardial infarction and cardiogenic shock.

He was started on vasopressors and O_2 and given opiates for pain.

Arrangements were made for cardiac catheterization and angiography. The angiography showed a left anterior descending occlusion, and the left ventricular angiogram demonstrated an ejection fraction of 50% with large area of apical and anterior akinesia and decreased septal motion.

The patient remained in cardiogenic shock, and an aortic balloon counter pulsation was started.

Despite all efforts and aggressive management of the shock, the patient had a cardiac arrest and was pronounced dead twenty-four hours after admission.

DISCUSSION

This case illustrates one of the most serious complications of an acute myocardial infarction—cardiogenic shock resulting from major impairment of contractile power of the left ventricle.

In the evaluation of individuals in shock, three different types must be considered:

- *Cardiogenic.* Defined as sustained low blood pressure, below 90 mm Hg for at least thirty minutes despite adequate preload. The clinical picture includes signs of low cardiac output, cool extremities, and often, altered level of consciousness. Most often caused by an acute myocardial infarction.

- *Hypovolemic.* Most commonly caused by blood or fluid loss resulting in volume depletions in excess of 15–30% of vascular volume. The volume depletion is accompanied by tachycardia, vasoconstriction, decreased urine production, and in extreme cases, mental status change.

- *Distributive.* The most common cause of distributive shock are anaphylaxis and neurological accidents. As opposed to other types of shock, cardiac output is increased and peripheral vascular resistance is decreased.

Below are some facts about cardiogenic shock:

- It is observed in 7.5% of patients with ST acute myocardial infarction elevation and in 2.5% of patients with non–ST segment elevation myocardial infarction (NSTEMI),
- Despite new treatments, in-hospital mortality continues to be as high as 70–80%.
- Diabetics are twice as likely to develop cardiogenic shock.
- Left ventricular dysfunction (LVD) is the most frequent cause of cardiogenic shock (74.5%). Other causes include acute mitral regurgitation (8.3%), ventricular septal rupture (4.6%), isolated right ventricular infarction (3.4%), and tamponade or cardiac rupture (1.7%).
- Around 60% of patients have triple vessel disease. Left main disease is encountered in 20%, and the left anterior descending artery (LAD) is the most frequently involved artery.
- The median time from the onset of infarction to shock development is 5.6 hours.

What are some of the most important pathophysiological changes that take place in an individual in cardiogenic shock?

- Ischemia due to decreased coronary perfusion leads to muscle hypoxia and necrosis, resulting in impaired myocardial contractility.
- Cardiac output is decreased because of the decreased and abnormal contractility.
- Arterial blood pressure is reduced (< 70mm Hg).
- The sympathetic system responds to the reduced blood pressure by increasing vasoconstriction and heart rate and protection of perfusion to critical areas.

- The hormonal system is also activated, leading to salt and water retention.
- There is a severe decrease in renal blood flow and urine production.
- Lactic acidosis and hypoxia develop. They will further compromise myocardial contractility.

The prognosis of cardiogenic shock is grave, both acutely and over a five-year period. Mortality at one year approximates 30% and at five years 70%.

TREATMENT

Treatment of cardiogenic shock includes the following:

- Aspirin and heparin, the initial treatment.
- Oxygen, determined by level of O_2 saturation.
- Morphine for treatment of pain. It also decreases the preload and may help cardiac function by small increase in contractility.
- Inotropes and vasopressors like dopamine or dobutamine (it may cause vasodilatation and hypotension) and catecholamines. Dopamine, an inotrope and a vasopressor, is preferred initially.
- Diuretics are added if pulmonary congestion is present but consider its impact on preload.
- Intra-aortic balloon pump (IABP) is required for stabilizing patients before reperfusion therapies.
  Intra-aortic balloon pump is a support strategy where a balloon is introduced and advanced to the descending aorta and connected to a pump that inflates during diastole. It increases coronary blood flow during diastole and decreases the afterload by lowering systemic vascular resistance during systole. The use of IABP has

reduced in-hospital mortality to 50%, when compared to those who did not have IABP (mortality 72%, P<0.0001).
- Reperfusion.
    - *Fibrinolytic therapy.* When used in patients with AMI without shock, it decreases shock onset. Timely intervention reduces the onset of shock since it is known that shock development occurs after six hours of presentation to the hospital. These six hours are crucial for institution of treatment and can play a role in the prevention of cardiogenic shock.
    - *Coronary angioplasty.* The American College of Cardiology / American Heart Association (ACC/AHA) guidelines recommend early revascularization for patients < seventy-five years of age with cardiogenic shock.
    - *Coronary bypass surgery.* Patients in cardiogenic shock undergoing emergency coronary artery bypass surgery have mortality rates of around 25% to 60%.

CASE 15 QUESTIONS

1. In a patient with sepsis and shock you would expect

    a. Peripheral vascular resistance is elevated
    b. Peripheral vascular resistance is decreased
    c. Urinary output is increased
    d. Pulmonary pressure is elevated

2. Placement of an intra-aortic balloon pump in a patient with an acute MI

    a. Increases systolic pressure
    b. Improves coronary flow
    c. Increases peripheral resistance
    d. Decreases stroke volume

3. In a patient with cardiogenic shock and lactic acidosis

    a. Cardiac contractility is increased
    b. Pulmonary circulation is affected
    c. Cardiac contractility is decreased
    d. Arterial pH is elevated

4. Intra-aortic balloon pump in patients with cardiogenic shock has

    a. Not changed prognosis
    b. Has decreased mortality
    c. Can be maintained for months
    d. Lowers diastolic pressure

5. Cardiogenic shock is

    a. More common in diabetics
    b. Indicate left circumflex occlusion

c. Seen only intraventricular septal rupture
d. Is contraindicated in acute mitral regurgitation

6. A patient with a GI bleed will go into hypovolemic shock when blood volume

    a. Decreases by 10%
    b. Decreases by 30%
    c. Decreases by 50%
    d. Decreases by 75%

CASE NO. 16: ACUTE MYOCARDIAL INFARCTION—HYPOTENSION

Mr. RB, a sixty-four-year-old retired military officer and schoolteacher, develops chest pain as he is walking uphill on the Eighteenth Fairway. He stops to rest, and the pain subsides. During the rest of the day, he suffers two brief episodes of chest pain that subside quickly and decides he should seek medical attention the next day.

That night, while resting, again develops the same chest pain—intense, precordial radiating to the shoulders and left arm.

His wife calls 911, and he is transported without haste to a nearby community hospital. Upon arrival to the ED, his vital signs are pulse 90 per minute, BP 80/60, and respiration 18x'. An ECG is obtained and is shown below.

The ECG on admission reveals marked ST elevation in leads 2, 3, AVF and depression leads AVR and V1 and V2. R to S ration in V1 exceeds 1. The ECG is diagnostic of an acute interior infarction

He was admitted to the coronary unit, and an angiogram and angioplasty were performed. For forty-eight hours, he remained hypotensive with a BP of 80/60.

His hemodynamic state was normalized, and he was discharged in seven days.

DISCUSSION

The case presents with an acute inferior myocardial infarction complicated with hypotension.

Why can someone with an acute MI become hypotensive? What are some of the pathophysiology?

A simple approach to a patient with hypotension and an acute myocardial infarction is as follows:

- *If hypotensive with an anterior infarction, hypotension is most often caused by a left ventricular contractility issue.*

- *If hypotensive with an inferior infarction, consider right ventricular involvement and a preload issue.*

In this case, hypotension may be related to right ventricular infarction extending from the infarction of the inferior wall of the left ventricle.

The electrocardiographic criteria to diagnose right ventricular involvement are

- ST depression V1 and V2, with high specificity
- Prominent R in V1 (R > S in V1)

Both criteria are present in this patient and in addition to the tall R in V1 (reciprocal to Q waves in leads v7-v8), which is very indicative of infarction of the posterior wall of the left ventricle.

Right ventricular (RV) myocardial infarction

- very rarely occurs alone and most often occurs in the setting of inferior wall myocardial infarction,
- complicates approximately 25% (range, 20%–60%) of inferior acute myocardial infarction, and
- is rare in anterior and lateral wall acute myocardial infarction.

THE PATHOPHYSIOLOGY

The right ventricle has two fundamental functions:

- ° To provide flow to the low pressure, low resistance right-side circulation
- ° To provide and control the preload of the left ventricle

Left ventricular filling pressure is dependent upon the patient's preload controlled by the right side of the circulation.

In a right ventricular infarction in the setting of an acute inferior infarction, hypotension causes a preload issue. Any agent that can lower preload (i.e., morphine) may further lower systemic blood pressure.

In this case, the clinical presentation is as follows:

- ST elevation myocardial infarction (STEMI) of the inferior wall
- Hypotension
- Jugular venous distension
- Electrocardiographic findings: ST segment elevation of greatest magnitude in lead 3 (compared with leads 2 and AVF), ST segment depression in lead V1 and depression in V2 (a very sensitive and specific criteria for right ventricular involvement). Recording precordial leads on the right side of the chest provides additional supportive data.

TREATMENT

Therapy, in addition to appropriate management for STEMI, relies largely on enhancing preload with intravenous fluid and judicious use of vasodilator medications.

Angioplasty with stent insertion or thrombolytic therapy are indicated therapies.

Patients with inferior wall STEMI and RV infarction have a markedly worse prognosis (both acute cardiovascular complications and death) compared with patients with isolated inferior wall STEMI.

This patient recovered well and was discharged on the eight hospital day.

CASE 16 QUESTIONS

1. Right ventricular involvement in an acute MI is usually associate with a lesion in the

    a. Left coronary
    b. Left circumflex
    c. Right coronary
    d. Left perforator

2. Right ventricular involvement will affect

    a. Preload
    b. Afterload
    c. Venous return
    d. Left coronary circulation

3. Administration of morphine sulfate may decrease

    a. Contractility
    b. Preload
    c. None of the above
    d. All of the above

4. In the presence of right ventricular involvement, the following is likely to be observed

    a. Elevated pulmonary pressure
    b. Elevated right ventricular pressure
    c. Elevated right atrial pressure
    d. Elevated pulmonary capillary pressure

5. Right ventricular infarction occurs in

    a. 25% of all infarcts
    b. 25% of all anterior infarcts
    c. 25% of all inferior infarcts
    d. 25% of all subendocardial (non-STMI)

CASE NO. 17: UNSTABLE ANGINA PECTORIS

RB, a sixty-five-year-old retired teacher, developed acute precordial chest pain while playing golf on a Saturday afternoon. He rested for a while, and the pain subsided. He recognized the pain immediately, since it was identical to the exercise angina pectoris he was having for at least a year and had gotten it treated. Because of the pain episode, he terminated the golf game and drove home.

That night, he woke up at 2:00 a.m. with a similar episode, but it was lasting longer and was only partially relieved with one sublingual nitroglycerin. Concerned, he summoned the rescue squad that transported him to a local university hospital nearby.

After initial laboratory work was performed, it was decided that a cardiac catheterization and coronary angiogram was necessary, and it was performed the following morning.

The ECG, obtained after arrival and while he was having pain, is shown below, showing ST segment depression in 1, AVL, and left precordial leads

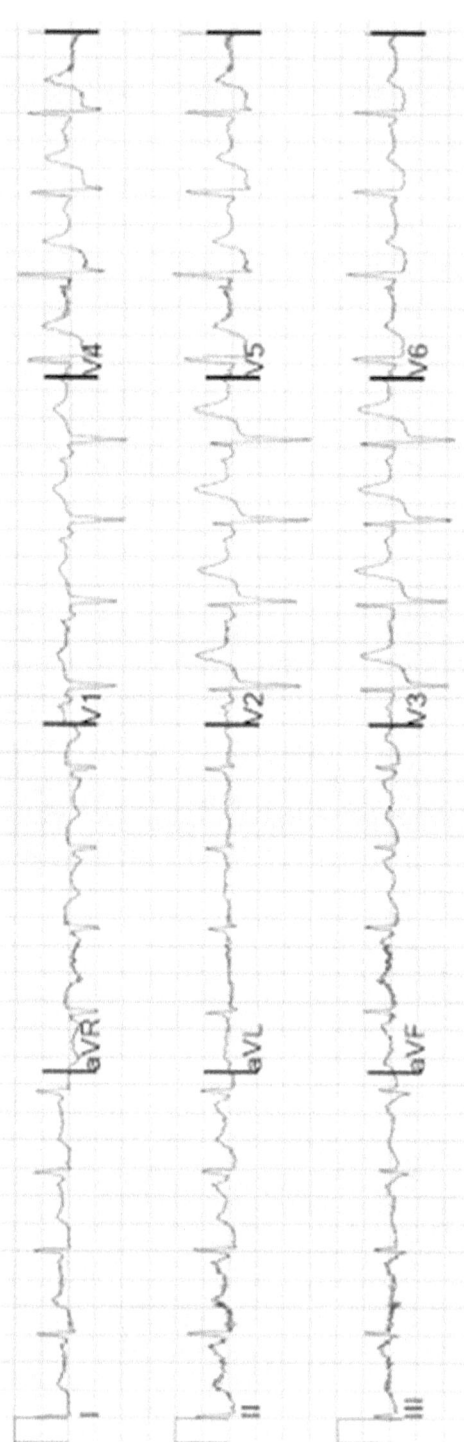

Fig 17.1

Further evaluation of his medical past history revealed that he had a strong family history—father had died of sudden death, brother had coronary disease, and sister had hypercholesterolemia. The patient had a history of moderate essential hypertension and type 2 diabetes.

Physical examination reveals an obese (300 lbs.) man in no distress. BP was 176/94, pulse 68. No cardiovascular findings were reported, and the remaining of the physical was noncontributory.

His biomarkers were normal.

Evaluation of his history, ECG, and angiographic data that revealed triple vessel disease with an 85% obstruction in the left anterior coronary prompted the decision to immediately perform coronary bypass surgery, and that was done a few hours later.

The patient recovered well.

DISCUSSION

The patient being discussed had exercise induced angina pectoris prior to the most recent episode. The clinical presentation on this occasion is quite different.

The development of chest pain at rest is one of the classical presentations of unstable angina.

There are three symptoms that should be clear warnings that exercise angina is now evolving and presenting with symptoms of unstable angina or an acute MI:

- Marked increase in the frequency of anginal chest pain
- Chest pain while resting

- Onset of nocturnal chest pain

Any of these symptoms require immediate attention since they represent a different set of pathophysiological changes.

What is the pathophysiology of unstable angina?

It includes the following:

- *Plaque rupture.* Plaque rupture often result in unstable angina or acute infarction.
  A plaque grows, macrophage, proteases, and neutrophil elastases within the plaque can increase instability of the plaque causing fissure mainly at the junction with the vessel wall. This will create a cascade of events leading to thrombosis and vasoconstriction.

- *Thrombosis.* Aggregation of platelets is caused by exposure to thromboxane and adenosine diphosphate leading to clot formation. Vaoconstriction is also caused by he production of thrombin that stabilizes the thrombi by converting fibrinogen to fibrin.
  Unstable angina, may involve a clot in flux forming and enlarging, chipping off, and embolizing.

- *Vasoconstriction.* Most patients with ACS have recurrent transient reduction in coronary blood supply because of vasoconstriction and thrombus formation at the site of atherosclerotic plaque rupture.
  Platelets release substances that promote vasoconstriction, and the combination of all—plaque rupture, thrombosis, and vasoconstriction—will eventually lead to death of myocardial tissue.

- *Supply-demand mismatch.* The supply-demand mismatch usually observed with exercise-induced angina will occur in unstable angina because of the further narrowing of the coronary caused by vasoconstriction and thrombus formation in the vessel lumen. This issue was discussed previously. Ischemia results from excessive demand or inadequate supply of oxygen, glucose, and free fatty acids.

Symptoms of unstable angina are similar to those of myocardial infarction (MI) and represent a true medical emergency that needs to be accompanied by hospitalization, diagnostic tests, and coronary angiography.

Electrocardiograms and serial cardiac biomarker assays are essential to make the diagnosis.

A coronary angiogram and ventricular angiogram are essential to determine the anatomy as well as ventricular function. The course of unstable angina is highly variable and potentially life-threatening; therefore, the initial treatment approach should use angioplasty with placements of stents or surgical management or a conservative medical management strategy.

Patients who present with new ST segment deviation ($\geq$ 1 mm) have a one-year death or an MI rate of 11%, compared with a rate of only 6.8% in patients with isolated T wave inversion.

TREATMENT

The management of unstable angina includes the use of

- Antiplatelet agents, lipid-lowering statin agents

- Cardiovascular antiplatelet agents (e.g., tirofiban, eptifibatide, and abciximab)
- Beta-blockers
- Anticoagulants
- Low-molecular-weight heparins
- Thrombin inhibitors
- Nitrates (e.g., nitroglycerin IV)
- Angiotensin-converting enzyme inhibitors

Having obtained the angiographic data, the decision must be made to proceed with angioplasty and stent insertion or coronary bypass surgery. In some cases, intensive medical management may be indicated.

CASE 17 QUESTIONS

1. Plaque rupture is essential to cause unstable angina. Plaque rupture is likely to be seen

    a. With calcified plaques
    b. With thick plaques
    c. With thrombosed plaques
    d. With thin plaques

2. Myocardial infarction occurs

    a. In thin plaques
    b. In calcified plaques
    c. In thick plaques
    d. In significant or insignificant plaques
    e. In plaques without thrombi

3. Vasoconstriction is

    a. Rare in acute coronary syndromes
    b. Is affected by platelets that release vasoconstricting substances
    c. Does not affect coronary diameter
    d. Occurs late in ACS process

4. In unstable angina

    a. No genetic factors exist
    b. Apolipoproteins have no role
    c. Polymorphisms in several matrix metalloproteinase (MMP) genes have been described
    d. Coronary supply is not affected

5. The diagnosis and management of unstable angina

    a. Can be done with ECGs alone
    b. Can be made with use of biomarkers alone
    c. Does not need and angiogram
    d. Needs Antiplatelet aggregation therapy

CASE NO. 18: ORTHOSTATIC HYPOTENSION IN A POST-MI HYPERTENSIVE PATIENT

Mr. RB is a sixty-seven-year-old retired schoolteacher with a past history of unstable angina who presents to the office in search for a second opinion. He was diagnosed as having severe hypertension and is currently taking three different medications for his hypertension. He reports that since the recent adjustments of the drugs, he has noted severe dizziness when he gets up in the morning, fearing that he is going to faint. These symptoms may repeat themselves during the day as he stands up abruptly.

Past history is remarkable for coronary artery disease, having undergone triple coronary bypass two years ago.

Physical examination is as follows:

BP is 190/70 supine and 160/76 standing. Pulse is 55x' supine and 80x' standing

Patient is 74 inches tall and weighs 290 pounds.

All arterial pulses are present, and no carotid bruits detected.

Cardiovascular examination reveals no cardiomegaly, and heart sounds are normal. No murmurs are present.

Remaining of the physical examination is unremarkable except for substantial obesity and very prominent abdominal girth.

DISCUSSION

In this case, the diagnosis of orthostatic hypotension is clear. The diagnostic criteria being used is a drop in systolic blood pressure of 20 mm Hg or 10 mm Hg of diastolic pressure when moving from the supine to the standing position.

What are the potential causes of orthostatic hypotension?

In this case, the most likely cause is the medications he is taking for the control of his hypertension.

When evaluating a patient with orthostatic hypotension one has to consider the possible causes that can be divided in neurogenic and non-neurogenic causes.

NEUROGENIC CAUSES

Neurogenic orthostatic hypotension can be due to neuropathy (e.g., diabetic neuropathy) or to central lesions (e.g., Parkinson's disease).

NON-NEUROGENIC CAUSES

Non-neurogenic causes include

- Cardiac diseases such as myocardial infarction or aortic stenosis
- Reduced intravascular volume (e.g., from dehydration,) and vasodilation
- Common drugs that cause orthostatic hypotension, like diuretics, alpha-adrenoceptor blockers for prostatic hypertrophy, antihypertensive drugs, and calcium channel blockers, levodopa, and tricyclic antidepressants

ORTHOSTATIC HYPOTENSION IN THE ELDERLY

The prevalence of orthostatic hypotension is high in the elderly and depends on the characteristics of the population studied, such as age, use of medications, and comorbidities known to be associated with this problem. Orthostatic hypotension is more common in institutionalized elderly people (up to 68%) than in those living in the community (6%).

How is blood pressure regulated?

Regulation of BP is a complex physiological function that depends on local as well as central mechanisms.

Local (peripheral) regulation primarily achieves a tight matching of regional blood flow to local metabolic needs. It occurs through locally produced mediators (autacoids), including eicosanoids, nitric oxide, endothelins, and tissue plasminogen activator.

Central regulation maintains control of BP through changes in cardiac output and vascular tone mediated by the autonomic nervous system.

- The sympathetic nervous system plays the predominant role in determining the level of arterial BP and the distribution of cardiac output.
- The parasympathetic nervous system is almost negligible in the regulation of vascular tone, and its effect occurs mainly via its negative chronotropic and inotropic effects.
- Central regulatory mechanisms control the sympathetic outflow to the cardiovascular system in both short- and long-term.

- Short-term reflex control of the sympathetic vasomotor activity is regulated by homeostatic feedback mechanisms, such as the baroreceptor and chemoreceptor reflexes. Central mechanisms also produce specific patterns of sympathetic activity according to different external stimuli or stresses.
- Long-term control depends on the interplay of several mechanisms, including
    - changes in the sympathetic vasomotor outflow,
    - renal control of extracellular volume,
    - pressure natriuresis, and
    - the activity of antagonistic "push-pull" systems, such as the kallikrein-kinin and renin-angiotensin-aldosterone systems.

What is the physiology of the upright posture?

Orthostatic stress is a common daily challenge for humans when posture changes from lying to standing or during prolonged quiet standing.

With the transition from the supine to the erect position, a gravitational shift of nearly five hundred milliliters of blood away from the chest to the distensible venous capacitance system below the diaphragm takes place. This results in a rapid decrease in central blood volume and a subsequent reduction of ventricular preload, stroke volume, and mean BP.

In the vascular system, a reference quantitative determinant of these changes is the venous hydrostatic indifference point (HIP), when pressure is independent of posture. The venous HIP is approximately at the diaphragmatic level and is significantly affected by venous compliance and muscular activity.

Upon standing, contractions of lower limb muscles, along with the presence of venous valves, provide an intermittent unidirectional flow, moving the venous HIP toward the right atrium. Respiration may also increase venous return because deep inspiration results in both a decline in thoracic pressure and an increase in intra-abdominal pressure, which lowers retrograde flow due to compression of both the iliac and femoral veins.

To provide an appropriate perfusion pressure to critical organs, an effective set of the neural regulatory system is promptly activated upon standing. The sympathetic nervous system is fast acting and primarily modulated by mechanoreceptors and, to a smaller degree, by chemoreceptors. Arterial baroreceptors (high-pressure receptors) are located in the carotid sinus and the aortic arch and—by conveying baroceptive impulses via carotid sinus and aortic depressor nerves to the brainstem, notably in the nucleus of the solitary tract—determine tonic inhibition of vasomotor centers. A sudden drop in BP in the carotid sinus and the aortic arch triggers baroreceptor-mediated compensatory mechanisms within seconds, resulting in increased heart rate, myocardial contractility, and peripheral vasoconstriction

In addition, the veno-arteriolar axon reflex results in constriction of arterial flow to the muscles, skin, and adipose tissue, leading to almost one-half of the increase in vascular resistance in the limbs upon standing. Ultimately, orthostatic stabilization is normally achieved in roughly one minute or less.

During prolonged quiet standing, transcapillary filtration in the subdiaphragmatic space further reduces central blood volume and cardiac output by approximately 15% to 20%. This transcapillary shift equilibrates after approximately thirty minutes of upright posture, which can result in a net fall in plasma volume of up to 10% over this time.

Continued upright posture results in activation of neuroendocrine mechanisms, such as the renin-angiotensin-aldosterone system, which may vary in intensity depending on the volume status.

The most important homeostatic response to prolonged orthostatic stress appears to be the carotid baroreflex-mediated increase of peripheral vascular resistance.

The inability of any one of these factors may result in a failure of the system to compensate for an initial or sustained postural challenge. This may produce a transient or persistent state of hypotension, which, in turn, can lead to symptomatic cerebral hypoperfusion and loss of consciousness, either in the early or late phase of orthostatic challenge

TREATMENT

Orthostatic hypotension is generally resolved with treatment of the underlying cause. In this case, adjustment of the antihypertensive drugs and instructions to take his medications in the evening was sufficient to eliminate the orthostasis.

In patients with chronic orthostatic hypotension, pharmacologic and nonpharmacologic treatments may be beneficial.

All patients with chronic orthostatic hypotension should be educated about their diagnosis and goals of treatment, which include improving orthostatic blood pressure without excessive supine hypertension, improving standing time, and relieving orthostatic symptoms.

NONPHARMACOLOGIC TREATMENT

Patients should do the following:

- Avoid large carbohydrate-rich meals (to prevent postprandial hypotension).

- Limit alcohol intake.

- Have adequate hydration. Older patients should consume a minimum of 1.25 to 2.50 L of fluid per day to balance expected twenty-four-hour urine losses. Water boluses (one 480-mL glass of tap water in one study and two 250-mL glasses of water in rapid succession in another study) have been shown to increase standing systolic blood pressure by more than 20 mm Hg for approximately two hours.

- Sodium may be supplemented by adding extra salt to food or taking 0.5- to 1.0-g salt tablets.

Lower extremity and abdominal binders may be beneficial

An exercise program focused on improving conditioning and teaching physical maneuvers to avoid orthostatic hypotension has proven to be beneficial.

PHARMACOLOGIC

In patients who do not respond adequately to nonpharmacologic therapy for orthostatic hypotension, medication may be indicated.

Fludrocortisone. Fludrocortisone, which is a synthetic mineralocorticoid, is considered first-line therapy for the treatment of orthostatic hypotension

Midodrine. Midodrine is a peripheral selective alpha-1 adrenergic agonist that significantly increases standing systolic blood pressure and improves symptoms in patients with neurogenic orthostatic hypotension.

Pyridostigmine (Mestinon). Pyridostigmine is a cholinesterase inhibitor that improves neurotransmission at acetylcholine-mediated neurons of the autonomic nervous system without worsening supine hypertension.

CASE 18 QUESTIONS

1. In the regulation of blood pressure after postural changes

    a. Sympathetic system is important
    b. Parasympathetic plays a critical role
    c. Volume changes to not play a role
    d. All of the above

2. The venous hydrostatic indifference point (HIP)

    a. Is fixed
    b. Is independent of muscle tone
    c. Is usually at the level of the diaphragm
    d. Is the same in the arterial system
    e. Is always constant

3. The referred drugs to treat orthostatic hypotension are

    a. SSRIs
    b. Mineralocorticoids
    c. Alpha-blockers
    d. Beta-blockers

4. A population frequently affected

    a. Diabetics
    b. Elderly
    c. Institutionalized
    d. All of the above
    e. None of the above

5. Heart rate will increase when a patient with orthostatic hypertension stands erect.

    a. True
    b. False

CASE NO 19: POST-MI VENTRICULAR TACHYCARDIA

Ms. BK, a 75 year old female reports to the ED complaining of shortness of breath, feeling like she is going to faint, and recognizing a very rapid heart rate.

Her past medical history is significant in that she had two myocardial infarctions in the last three years and, in the last few months, twice visited the ED with shortness of breath and rapid heart rate that was diagnosed as episodes of ventricular tachycardia and treated accordingly.

Physical examination is as follows:

BP 90/60, rate 165x', respiration 18x'

Cardiovascular examination reveals normal JVP and arterial pulses.

Apical impulse is slightly displaced to the left.

Auscultation: normal S1 and S2, S4 and soft S3 at the apex. Short, mid-frequency early pansystolic murmur at the apex compatible with mild mitral regurgitation.

ECG obtained at arrival to the ED.

This ECG shows Ventricular tachycardias with a fusion beat, one of the diagnostic criteria (+ wide QRS)

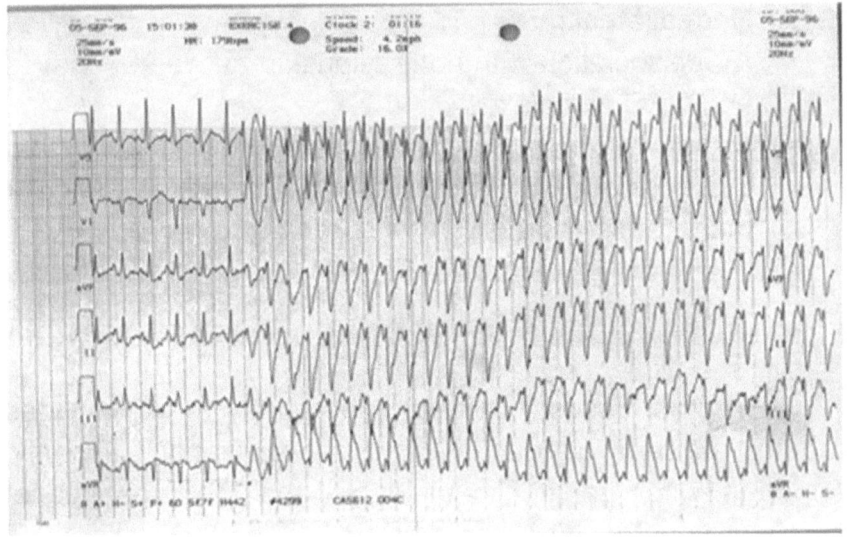

Fig. 33.1. ECG shows a ventricular rate of 150X' and wide QRS complexes compatible with ventricular tachycardia originating in the left ventricle.

DISCUSSION

Ventricular tachycardia (VT) or ventricular fibrillation (VF) cause most of the sudden cardiac deaths in the United States, at an estimated rate of approximately 300,000 deaths per year.

VT refers to any rhythm faster than 100 (or 200 beats per minute) with three or more irregular beats in a row, arising distal to the bundle of His. The rhythm may arise from working ventricular myocardium, the distal conduction system, or both.

Electrocardiographic recognition of ventricular tachycardia is based on the following criteria:

- Ventricular rate ranging between 100 and 180

- Abnormal QRS morphology with a duration greater than 0.10 seconds
- Normal atrial rate
- AV dissociation with no relationship between P waves and QRS complexes
- Fusion beats occurring when a supraventricular beat with normal QRS morphology merges with a ventricular tachycardia complex

ELECTROPHYSIOLOGY OF VENTRICULAR TACHYCARDIA

In most cases, the electrophysiology of VT includes reentry, namely conduction and repolarization disparity, opportunity for unidirectional block, and the presence of premature ventricular complexes (PVCs) as the initiator. VT can readily degenerate into ventricular fibrillation (VF), which almost always results into sudden death. The propensity for VT-to-VF degeneration is greatly influenced by the degree of left ventricular (LV) dysfunction.

In a subset of patients with LV dysfunction from cardiomyopathy, the reentry is through specialized bundle branches. This VT is called bundle branch reentry VT (BBR-VT). This distinction is important, because BBR-VT is curable with catheter ablation (usually of the right bundle branch). However, depending on the severity of underlying LV function, these patients may also benefit from an implantable defibrillator.

There are several other types of VT:

- Idiopathic VT can be present in healthy myocardium or ventricles with minimal abnormalities. It is believed to be caused by automaticity and/or triggered activity and is likely to self-terminate. It rarely degenerates into VF.

Idiopathic VT resulting from increased automaticity often originates in the right ventricular outflow tract or from the fascicles of the cardiac conduction system.

- Two subset of patients with no structural heart disease but who are still at risk for sudden death are

    - Long QT syndrome (to be discussed in a separate case)

    - *Brugada syndrome.* Brugada syndrome is characterized by the specific ECG pattern of right bundle branch block and ST segment elevation in the precordial leads, most commonly V1–V3 without any structural abnormality of the heart. It causes idiopathic polymorphic VT or VF and carries a high risk for sudden cardiac death. Brugada syndrome is inherited in an autosomal dominant fashion.

Both syndromes involve abnormality in repolarization, either from potassium-channel defect, sodium-channel defect, or both. Typically, there is a family history of sudden death at a very young age (less than forty years old).

VT can also be seen in conditions that create myocardial scars, such as the following:

- *Dilated cardiomyopathy.* Its genetic basis involve mutations in genes coding for proteins that make up cardiac sarcomeres, including actin, myosin, and troponin. Genes such as *PSEN1* and *PSEN2* have been implicated in dilated cardiomyopathy. Most familial dilated cardiomyopathies are inherited in an autosomal dominant fashion. Autosomal recessive inheritance has been described in mutations of the *TNNI3* gene, which encodes troponin.

- Hypertrophic cardiomyopathy

- *Arrhythmogenic right ventricular dysplasia (ARVD).* ARVD is characterized by replacement of the free wall of the right ventricle. This disorder frequently results in sustained VT, which may degrade into VF. The genetics of ARVD are extremely heterogeneous. It is inherited in an autosomal dominant fashion.

Other causes of ventricular tachycardia include the following:

- *Chagas disease.* Endemic in some regions of South America, this is caused by the *Trypanosoma cruzi*. It causes diseases of the esophagus and colon and very commonly causes a dilated cardiomyopathy, ventricular aneurysms, and ventricular tachycardia.

- *Surgical incisions in the ventricle.* The scar tissues can be the origin of recurrent VT.

- *Electrolyte deficiencies* (e.g., hypokalemia, hypocalcemia, and hypomagnesemia).

- *Systemic diseases that affect the myocardium* such as sarcoidosis, amyloidosis, systemic lupus erythematosus, hemochromatosis, and rheumatoid arthritis

- *Sympathomimetic agents* such as IV inotropes and illicit drugs such as methamphetamine or cocaine.

- *Digitalis toxicity.*

- *Drugs that prolong the QT interval* (see next case) such as class IA and class III antiarrhythmics, and other drugs including azithromycin, levofloxacin, and many others that may cause a ventricular tachycardia with a well-defined electrocardiographic morphology called torsades de pointes. Persons with this syndrome are predisposed to episodes of polymorphic VT. These episodes can be self-limited, resulting in syncope, or they may transition into VF and thus can cause sudden cardiac death. (Further discussion in a subsequent case.)

- *Drugs that slow conduction velocity,* such as halothane and class IA and IC antiarrhythmics).

- *Catecholamine polymorphic ventricular tachycardia.* Ventricular tachycardia can be induced by exercise or emotional stress.

What are the mechanisms and consequences of ventricular tachycardia?

Ventricular tachycardia is caused by electrical reentry or abnormal automaticity. Myocardial scarring from any process increases the likelihood of electrical reentrant circuits. These circuits generally include a zone where normal electrical propagation is slowed by a scar. Ventricular scar formation from a prior myocardial infarction (MI) is the most common cause of sustained monomorphic VT.

The hemodynamic consequences of ventricular tachycardia are very much influenced by the ventricular rate and the lack of effective atrial-ventricular coordination. During VT, cardiac output is reduced as a consequence of decreased ventricular filling time from the rapid heart rate and lack of properly timed or coordinated atrial contraction, a substantial contributor to end-diastolic volume and stroke volume. If the tachycardia induces myocardial ischemia, it may also contribute to decreased cardiac output. Diminished cardiac output may result in diminished myocardial perfusion, worsening inotropic response, The combination of all these factors may lead to ventricular fibrillation (VF), resulting in sudden death.

TREATMENT

Treatment should be based on the hemodynamic state of the patient.

- **Unstable patients** (hypotensive, shock, myocardial ischemia) with monomorphic VT should be immediately treated with synchronized direct current (DC) cardioversion.
- **Stable patients** with adequate organ perfusion and without signs or symptoms of hemodynamic compromise. The treatment will depends on whether the VT is monomorphic or polymorphic.

Patients with monomorphic VT and normal left ventricular function can be treated with intravenous (IV) procainamide, lidocaine, or sotalol.

Mounting evidence indicates that amiodarone should not be the first-line antiarrhythmic for stable VT, because its effects on myocardial conduction and refractoriness are gradual in onset. If medical therapy is unsuccessful, synchronized cardioversion should be used.

Radiofrequency ablation of the area of myocardium where the arrhythmia originates is a modern method of treatment of recurrent VT.

Insertion of a permanent defibrillator is important in patients with recurrent ventricular tachycardia or episode of ventricular fibrillation.

CASE 19 QUESTIONS

1. Ventricular tachycardia will show

    a. Fusion beats
    b. Broad QRS complexes
    c. AV dissociation
    d. All of the above

2. Ventricular tachycardia

    a. Originates in the right ventricle
    b. Originates in the left ventricle
    c. All of the above
    d. None of the above

3. If a patient has scarring of the left ventricle

    a. Ventricular tachycardia is caused by increased automaticity
    b. Ventricular tachycardia is caused by reentry
    c. Will respond only to cardioversion
    d. Can only be treated with lidocaine

4. In patients with ventricular tachycardia

    a. QT interval will always be prolonged
    b. There will always be serious hemodynamic changes
    c. Fusion beats cannot be seen
    d. None of the above
    e. All of the above

5. Which of the following can cause ventricular tachycardia?

    a. Sarcoidosis
    b. Digitalis
    c. Hypokalemia
    d. All of the above
    e. None of the above

CARDIOMYOPATHIES

HEART FAILURE

CASE NO. 20: POSTPARTUM HEART FAILURE— DILATED CARDIOMYOPATHY

DP, a thirty-two-year-old female on her twenty-eighth week of pregnancy, is referred to a cardiologist because of increasing shortness of breath while walking. She describes that in the last few weeks, she has not been able to walk more than two blocks, having to stop to regain her breath. On further questioning, she indicates waking up a couple of nights short of breath and now has to sleep on two pillows. She has noted swelling of feet and ankles that initially thought were related to the pregnancy

Her past medical history is noncontributory. She is on her third pregnancy, and the previous two were uncomplicated with normal deliveries.

Cardiovascular examination reveals BP 110/70, pulse 94 per minute, and respiration 18 per minute.

Cardiovascular examination demonstrates the following:

- Jugular veins slightly distended.
- Apical impulse slightly displaced to the left with a palpable S3.
- S1 is soft and S2 normal.
- Loud S3 at apex.
- Grade 2/6 pansystolic murmur at the apex.
- Extremities show 2+ pitting edema.

Remaining physical examination is unremarkable except for the findings of pregnancy.

Chest x-ray shows a large cardia image, and the echocardiogram demonstrates a decreased ejection fraction and a dilated left ventricle

DISCUSSION

The recent evidence of heart failure, in a young, otherwise healthy female in the last trimester of pregnancy, suggests peripartum cardiomyopathy (PPCM), a form of dilated cardiomyopathy, that typically appears between the last month of pregnancy and up to six months postpartum.

PPCM is clinically similar to other forms of dilated cardiomyopathy and has similar pathophysiological consequences. Peripartum cardiomyopathy involves primary systolic dysfunction, decreased left ventricular ejection fraction (EF) and increased risk of atrial and ventricular arrhythmias, thromboembolism, and sudden cardiac death.

PPCM may be slightly more prevalent among older multipara women. A quarter to a third of PPCM patients are young women in their first pregnancy.

Postpartum cardiomyopathy begins with an unknown trigger that initiates an inflammatory process in the heart, resulting in damage to myocardial cells and the formation of scar tissue. This results in an impaired contractile function and a decrease in cardiac output. The initial inflammatory process appears to cause an autoimmune or immune dysfunctional process, which in turn fuels the initial inflammatory process. Progressive loss of heart muscle cells leads to eventual heart failure.

The cause of PPCM remains unknown, though some theories suggest a cardiotropic virus, autoimmunity or immune system dysfunction, or toxins that serve as triggers to immune system dysfunction. It is estimated that the incidence of PPCM in the United States is between 1 in 1,300 to 4,000 live births. While it can affect women of all races, it is more prevalent in some countries, occurring at rates of one in 1,000 live births in South African Bantus and as high as one in 300 in Haiti.

As reported in the case discussed above, patients often complain of orthopnea, pitting edema, cough, frequent nighttime urination, excessive weight gain during the last month of pregnancy, palpitations, and atypical chest pain.

Early detection and treatment are critically important since delays in diagnosis and treatment of PPCM are associated with increased morbidity and mortality.

What are the pathophysiological changes associated with dilated cardiomyopathy such as peripartum cardiomyopathy?

The discussion that follows is applicable to all cases of dilated cardiomyopathy, secondary to any of the causes listed below:

The hemodynamic changes include the following:

- The initial impact is impairment in the myocardial contractile power, manifested by a decrease in the velocity of myocardial contraction.
- The abnormalities in the myocardium will lead to ventricular dilatation and changes in the geometry of the ventricle. These changes can be diffused or localized, creating areas of hypokinesia or akinesia.
- The alteration of ventricular geometry and dilatation disrupts the apex to the base pattern of contractility and also increases wall tension as a result of the increased diameter of the ventricle, facilitating further dilatation and associated hypertrophy.

- The impaired contractility will lower cardiac output and stroke volume.
- Compensatory mechanisms take place in an effort to maintain homeostasis, especially to maintain cardiac output. These mechanisms include the following:
    - Increased sympathetic response that will
        - increase heart rate to maintain stable cardiac output and
        - vasoconstriction to compensate for the decrease in systolic pressure caused by the decreased contractility.
    - Activate the renin-angiotensin axis that will result in fluid retention and vasoconstriction.
    - Increased atrial pressure and resulting increase in pulmonary pressures in order to sustain preload.
    - Atrial dilatation will cause increased production of antidiuretic peptides that will cause fluid retention.
    - Regional flow redistribution necessary to sustain normal flow to brain, kidney, and other critical systems.
- Ventricular dilatation will cause dilatation of the AV rings and a resulting mitral regurgitation that is deleterious to normal hemodynamics. Same thing could happen to the right ventricle causing tricuspid regurgitation.

What can cause a dilated cardiomyopathy?

Dilated cardiomyopathy can have many different etiologies and could be divided in several categories, although in many cases, no cause is apparent.

- *Ischemic cardiomyopathy*. Multiple episodes of coronary vasoconstriction or the presence of coronary disease leads to multiple ischemic episodes causing repetitive damage to the myocardium with cell necrosis that could lead to dilatation of the ventricle.
- *Infections*
    - Sequelae of acute viral myocarditis, such as with Coxsackie B virus and other enteroviruses possibly mediated through an immunologic mechanism
    - Chagas disease, due to *Trypanosoma cruzi*— the most common infectious cause of dilated cardiomyopathy in Latin America
    - HIV
    - Other viral infections
- *Toxic*
    - Alcohol abuse (alcoholic cardiomyopathy), although the cause-and-effect relationship with alcohol alone is debated.
    - Stimulants. Cocaine. Coronary vasoconstriction caused by cocaine results in myocardial ischemia or infarction as well as systemic vasoconstriction. While most cases of cocaine-related cardiomyopathy have proved to be reversible, others have resulted in permanent cardiac dysfunction or death.
    - Nonalcoholic toxic insults include
        - chemotherapeutic agents, in particular doxorubicin (Adriamycin), and cobalt.[4]
- *Hyperthyroidism* and chronic uncontrolled tachycardia.
- *Genetic*. About 25–35% of cardiomyopathies have a familial form with most mutations affecting genes encoding cytoskeletal proteins or affect other proteins involved in contraction. The disease is genetically

heterogeneous, and the most common form is an autosomal dominant pattern.
- *Muscular dystrophy*

Dilated cardiomyopathies are more common in African Americans than in Caucasians, but it may occur in any patient population.

TREATMENT

Treatment for PPCM and other dilated cardiomyopathies is similar to treatment of congestive heart failure, including the use of diuretics, beta-blockers, and angiotensin-converting enzyme inhibitor (ACE-I). If EF is less than 35%, anticoagulation is indicated, since there is a greater risk of developing left ventricular thrombi and subsequent embolization.

PPCM carres a good prognosis. the survival rate is 98% or better, improving dramatically with proper treatment with over 50% of patients having an ejection fraction greater than 55%.

If severe symptoms persist, more aggressive therapy is indicated, and in few cases, cardiac transplantation is necessary. If EF is below 55%left subsequent pregnancies should be avoided since the risk for recurrence of heart failure is approximately 21%.

CASE 20 QUESTIONS

1. In a twenty-eight-year-old with dilated cardiomyopathy

    a. Wall stress increases
    b. Ventricular volume is normal
    c. End systolic volume is decreased
    d. Myocardial O_2 consumption decreases

2. Cocaine can cause cardiomyopathy because of

    a. Toxic properties of cocaine
    b. Immune reaction
    c. Repetitive coronary vasoconstriction
    d. Hypotension

3. Which of the following does not cause a dilated cardiomyopathy?

    a. *Trypanosoma cruzi*
    b. HIV
    c. Syphilis
    d. Coxsackievirus

4. The causes of cardiomyopathies are multiple. One of the following facts is correct:

    a. Around 60% are a familial form
    b. The most common are recessive patterns
    c. Duchenne muscular dystrophy is X-linked
    d. Mitochondrial inheritance is not linked to cardiomyopathies

5. Postpartum cardiomyopathy

    a. Has a poor prognosis
    b. Is more common in southern Europe

c. More common in older women
   d. Very common in Haiti

6. Postpartum cardiomyopathy

   a. Incidence in US is one per 1,300 live births
   b. With appropriate therapy, the survival rate is 98% or better
   c. Subsequent pregnancy should not be avoided
   d. Anticoagulation is not indicated
   e. Cardiac transplantation will always be needed

CASE NO. 21: HYPERTENSION—DIASTOLIC HEART FAILURE

A seventy-five-year-old retired physician is referred to a cardiologist because his increasing shortness of breath results in decreasing exercise tolerance. He also admits that in the last six months, he has noted that shortness of breath appears when climbing stairs or walking at a fast pace on level ground. The symptoms have increased in the last couple of months, and it has limited its exercise capacity.

He reports a long history of essential hypertension diagnosed fifteen years ago and treated with diuretics and calcium channel with good results. The major issue was compliance. During these years, he went for protracted periods of time not taking his medications regularly, and in the meantime, he gained twenty pounds and continued to smoke a pack a day.

He denies episodes of exercise-related chest pain. Physical examination results with BP at 170/90, pulse 80x', and respiration 16x'.

Cardiovascular examination shows a slightly sustained apical impulse, and cardiac auscultation reveals a loud S4.

All peripheral pulses are normal.

The rest of the examination is unremarkable.

DISCUSSION

This case illustrates what happens when there is a substantial decrease in cardiac compliance as a result of left ventricular hypertrophy caused by long-term essential hypertension.

We will discuss two important topics, hypertension and diastolic heart failure resulting from the concentric left ventricular hypertrophy

DIASTOLIC HEART FAILURE

The pathophysiological changes that ensue after years developing hypertrophy and impacting compliance are as follows:

- Left ventricular end-diastolic pressure rises despite a normal contractility.

- The elevation of end-diastolic pressure leads to elevation of pulmonary capillary pressure, and if high enough, it will result in transudate fluid entering the pulmonary alveoli. This will eventually cause pulmonary edema.

- Cardiac output is lower than normal.

- Ejection fraction is often normal.

- Complete left ventricular filling is essential to maintain maximum cardiac output, and for that, the presence of normal sinus rhythm and its late diastolic contribution to ventricular filling is important.

- Diastolic function is determined by the relative end diastolic volume in relation to end-diastolic pressure and is therefore independent of left ventricular systolic function.

Diastolic dysfunction and **diastolic heart failure** are two different entities.

A patient is said to have **diastolic dysfunction** if signs and symptoms of heart failure are present, but the left ventricular ejection fraction is normal or has an elevated BNP level in the presence of normal ejection fraction.

Generally, **diastolic dysfunction** is a chronic process. When this chronic condition is well tolerated by an individual and no specific treatment may be indicated but therapy should be directed at the root cause.

Echocardiography is used to diagnose **diastolic dysfunction** since decreased ventricular compliance will increase of the "a" amplitude reversing "E/A" ratio.

Diastolic dysfunction is better tolerated if the atrium is able to pump blood into the ventricles in a coordinated fashion. This does not occur in atrial fibrillation (AF) where there is no coordinated atrial activity, and the left ventricle loses around 20% of its output.

Diastolic dysfunction is a common finding in the elderly otherwise healthy and asymptomatic.

Diastolic heart failure describes a clinical syndrome that can be caused by

- aging,
- myocardial ischemia,
- hypertension, and
- aortic stenosis.

The diagnosis of **diastolic heart failure** remains imprecise and is narrowly defined as "heart failure with normal systolic function" and a left ventricular ejection fraction of 60% or more).

In this case, two of the consequences of arterial hypertension that we will briefly discuss.

HYPERTENSION

Normal levels of blood pressure are systolic 120–129 mm Hg and/or diastolic 80–84 mm Hg. Optimal levels are systolic lower than 120 mm Hg and diastolic lower than 80 mm Hg, and high normal is a systolic of 130–139 mm Hg and/or diastolic 85–89 mm Hg.

What is the definition of hypertension?

The diagnosis of hypertension varies according to the age of the individual, since blood pressure, both systolic and diastolic, will increase with age and, as shown below, is influenced by race and gender.

The most recently accepted criteria to define hypertension are as follows:

> *Grade 1:* Systolic 140–159 mm Hg and/or diastolic 90–99 mm Hg
> *Grade 2*: Systolic 160–179 mm Hg or greater and/or diastolic 100–109 mm Hg
> *Grade 3*: Systolic 180 mm Hg or greater and/or diastolic 110 mm Hg or greater
> *Isolated systolic hypertension*: 140 mm Hg or greater and diastolic lower than 90 mm Hg

What are the most common causes of hypertension?

Hypertension can be broadly subdivided into primary and secondary hypertension.

ESSENTIAL HYPERTENSION

Also called **primary hypertension** or **idiopathic hypertension**, has no identifiable cause. It is the most common type of hypertension, affecting 95% of hypertensive patients.

Some important concepts

- It tends to be familial

- is likely to be the consequence of an interaction between environmental and genetic factors.

- Prevalence of essential hypertension increases with age,

- individuals with relatively high blood pressure at younger ages are at increased risk for the subsequent development of hypertension.

The diagnosis of hypertension is made when the average of 2 or more diastolic BP measurements on at least 2 subsequent visits is ≥ 90 mm Hg or when the average of multiple systolic BP readings on 2 or more subsequent visits is consistently ≥ 140 mm Hg. Individuals with high normal BP tend to maintain pressures that are above average for the general population and are at greater risk for development of definite hypertension.

Transient elevations of blood pressure can be caused by multiple circumstances most likely related to stress. White coat hypertension is a classic example and is related to the stress associated with visiting a physician office.

SECONDARY HYPERTENSION

A number of diseases can cause associated hypertension

Renal causes

- *Renovascular hypertension* often caused by a stenosis of a renal artery that decreases renal.
- **Polycystic kidney disease**. This causes multiple cysts, with concurrent development of hypertension and often leads to renal failure.
- *Chronic* **glomerulonephritis**
- **Endocrine disorders**
    - Hyperaldosteronism (Conn's syndrome)—idiopathic hyperaldosteronism, Liddle's syndrome (also called pseudoaldosteronism), and glucocorticoid remediable aldosteronism
    - Hyperparathyroidism
    - Hyperthyroidism
    - Hypothyroidism
    - Juxtaglomerular cell tumor,
    - *Neurogenic hypertension*—excessive secretion of norepinephrine and epinephrine
        - Pheocromocytoma tha results in an excessive secretion of norepinephrine and epinephrine, which promotes vasoconstriction
    - *Primary* aldosteronism
        - Renal cell carcinoma—all of which may produce renin
        - Wilms' tumor

- **Other causes of secondary hypertension**

    - Drugs. In particular, alcohol, nasal decongestants with adrenergic effects, NSAIDs, MAOIs, adrenoceptor stimulants, and combined methods of hormonal contraception (those containing ethinylestradiol) can cause hypertension while in use.
    - *Herbal* or natural products, such as St. John's wort and licorice.
    - Hormonal contraceptives.
    - Neurofibromatosis.
    - Neurologic disorders.
    - Nicotine *use*.
    - Obstructive sleep apnea.
    - *Perioperative hypertension.*
    - Pregnancy.
    - Scleroderma.
    - Steroid *use*.
    - White coat hypertension.
    - *Arsenic exposure.*

What is the influence of age, gender, and ethnicity?

The prevalence of essential hypertension by age and ethnicity is as follows:

Age	Men	Women
20–34	11%	7%
35–44	25%	19%
45–54	37%	34%
55–64	54%	53%
65–74	64%	69%
> 75	67%	78%

Table 20.1

The influence or ethnicity is important, and the prevalence of hypertension according to race is as follows:

	Men	Women
African-American	43%	45%
White	34%	31%
Mexican	28%	29%
All	34%	33%

Table 20.2

What is the pathophysiology of essential hypertension?

The two main factors that will determine blood pressure levels are

- cardiac output and
- peripheral vascular resistance.

In the young, cardiac output is high, and with aging, there is a gradual decrease in output with a concomitant increase in peripheral vascular resistance.

Hypertension is produced by alteration in the regulation of these factors. Three theories have been proposed to explain this:

- An overactive renin-angiotensin system leads to vasoconstriction and retention of sodium and water. The increase in blood volume leads to hypertension.
- An overactive sympathetic nervous system leads to increased stress response with increased vascular resistance.

Although factors regulating blood pressure are well-known, the precise etiology of essential hypertension is not known but is clearly a combination of genetic, environmental, socioeconomic, and cultural components.

TREATMENT

Secondary hypertension requires management of the primary cause causing the blood pressure elevation.

The management of essential hypertension is based on lowering either output or resistance, and numerous drugs are available.

NONPHARMACOLOGIC THERAPY

- Dietary changes

    Salt restriction. The American Heart Association recommends that the average daily consumption of sodium chloride should not exceed six grams; this may lower BP by 2–8 mm Hg.

    Dietary potassium, calcium, and magnesium consumption have an inverse association with BP. Lower intake of these elements potentiates the effect of sodium on BP. Oral potassium supplementation may lower both systolic and diastolic BP. Calcium and magnesium supplementation have elicited small reductions in BP.

    Alcohol consumption. Daily alcohol intake should be restricted to less than 1 ounce of ethanol in men and 0.5 ounce in women.

Weight loss and exercise. Weight reduction may lower blood pressure by 5–20 mm Hg per ten kilograms of weight loss in a patient whose weight is more than 10% of the ideal body weight. Regular aerobic physical activity can facilitate weight loss, decrease BP, and reduce the overall risk of cardiovascular disease. Blood pressure may be lowered by 4–9 mm Hg with moderately intense physical activity. These activities include brisk walking for 30 minutes a day, 5 days per week. More intense workouts of 20–30 minutes, 3–4 times a week, may also lower BP and have additional health benefits.

PHARMACOLOGIC THERAPY

Angiotensin-converting enzyme inhibitors / angiotensin receptor blockers, calcium channel blockers, and thiazide diuretics are equally efficacious in hypertensive nonblack populations, whereas calcium channel blockers and thiazide diuretics are favored in black patients. Beta-blockers are no longer considered first-line therapy for hypertension.

Over 50% of patients with hypertension will require more than one drug for blood pressure control. In stage 1 hypertension, a single agent is generally sufficient to reduce BP, whereas in stage 2, a multidrug approach may be needed.

CASE 21 QUESTIONS

1. Diastolic heart failure can be seen in

    a. Coxsackie myocarditis
    b. Postpartum myocarditis
    c. Aortic stenosis
    d. Mitral regurgitation

2. In diastolic heart failure

    a. End-diastolic volume is elevated
    b. Compliance is increased
    c. End-systolic volume is high
    d. Ventricular compliance is decreased

3. Diastolic dysfunction

    a. Is common in the elderly
    b. Increases ventricular compliance
    c. Ejection fraction is always abnormal
    d. End-diastolic pressure is always low

4. In a patient with diastolic dysfunction

    a. Ejection fraction is low
    b. Symptoms of heart failure can be absent
    c. BNP is elevated
    d. End-systolic pressure is low

5. In a patient with diastolic dysfunction who develops atrial fibrillation

    a. Symptoms will improve
    b. End-systolic volume will not change
    c. End-diastolic pressure will increase
    d. Lack of atrial contraction may worsen symptoms

CASE NO. 22: RESTRICTIVE CARDIOMYOPATHY

A sixty-five-year-old is referred to a cardiologist with a history of progressive shortness of breath, swelling in lower extremities, palpitations, and two brief fainting episodes. The patient has a longstanding history of rheumatoid arthritis. He has no history of diabetes or hypercholesterolemia. He recently retired as a school principal and has been sedentary most of his adult life.

Physical examination is as follows:

BP = 100/60, P = 100x', R = 16x'

No evidence of cardiomegaly.

On auscultation, a loud S3 is heard. No heart murmurs detected.

Substantial pitting edema in lower extremities.

DISCUSSION

Restrictive cardiomyopathy (RCM) is a rare disease of the myocardium and is the least common of the cardiomyopathies, accounting for only 5% of all primary myocardial diseases.

This disease may be idiopathic or associated with other diseases, such as

- amyloidosis,
- hemosiderosis, or
- endomyocardial fibrosis.

In this case, amyloidosis is the most likely cause of the cardiomyopathy since it results in the deposition of the amyloid protein in the myocardium.

On the basis of the amyloid protein composition, amyloidosis is classified into four different varieties as follows:

- Primary or myeloma-related amyloidosis.
- Secondary amyloidosis. Secondary to chronic diseases such as tuberculosis or rheumatoid arthritis.
- Senile amyloidosis. Amyloid infiltration of the heart is common in the elderly population (systemic senile amyloidosis) and may impair diastolic-filling properties.
- Familial amyloidosis.

Other causes of restrictive cardiomyopathy include the following:

- Radiation fibrosis. This complication of radiotherapy, like pericardial constriction, is evident several years after treatment. Differentiating between constriction and restriction may be particularly difficult in these patients because the two conditions may coexist.
- Metastatic malignancies
- Anthracycline toxicity
- Eosinophilic cardiomyopathy and endomyocardial fibrosis. This eosinophilic cardiomyopathy, also known as Loeffler endocarditis, is associated with dense endomyocardial fibrosis and intraventricular thrombus formation.

In the early stages of the disease, typical restrictive hemodynamics may not be evident; however, in more advanced cases, typical restrictive hemodynamics are more likely.

The prognosis appears to be worse in children than in adults. Children require relatively high filling pressures for maintenance of systolic output, and the therapeutic margin between volume depletion (leading to low output) and volume overload (leading to congestive heart failure) is narrow.

Thromboembolic complications may occur.

The principal pathophysiological changes are as follows:

- Diastolic filling of the ventricles is limited.
- Contractility and wall thickness remain normal.
- The pressure/volume loop will show a rapid rise in pressure with small changes in ventricular volume.
- The change in pressure will end at the completion of rapid ventricular filling.
- Cardiac output will be decreased, accompanied by the other compensatory changes (increased heart rate and peripheral vascular resistance, elevated end-diastolic pressures, and atrial pressure, etc.)
- Hemodynamically, it has similarities with constrictive pericarditis characterized by a square root sign of the diastolic pressure curve seen in the atrial as well as ventricular curves.
- Reduced ventricular compliance.
- Ventricles cannot fill adequately at normal diastolic pressures.
- Reduced left ventricular filling volume leads to reduced stroke volume and low cardiac output, resulting in symptoms and signs of left-side failure, right-side

failure, or both because it affects both ventricles and presents with dominant right-side fluid retention.
- Complete heart block may result from fibrosis of the sinoatrial or the atrioventricular nodes.
- Mitral and tricuspid regurgitation may develop as a result of endocardial fibrosis.

TREATMENT

When this chronic condition is well tolerated, no specific treatment may be indicated.

If symptomatic, therapy should be directed at the root cause of the stiff left ventricle, with potential causes and aggravating factors like high blood pressure and diabetes treated appropriately.

Beta-blockers could be used as they induce bradycardia and give more time for ventricular filling. There is some evidence that calcium channel blocker drugs may be of benefit in reducing ventricular stiffness

CASE 22 QUESTIONS

1. The classical hemodynamic finding in restrictive cardiomyopathy is

    a. Low cardiac output
    b. Low end-diastolic pressure
    c. Square root sign in ventricular pressure
    d. Tachycardia

2. The differential diagnosis includes

    a. Obstructive cardiomyopathy
    b. Pericarditis
    c. Dilated cardiomyopathy
    d. Congestive heart failure

3. Multiple blood transfusions may lead to a restrictive cardiomyopathy because of

    a. Deposits of amyloid
    b. Deposits of hemoglobin
    c. Myocardial fibrosis
    d. Deposits of iron

4. In restrictive cardiomyopathy

    a. Ventricular filling ends early
    b. End diastolic pressure is low
    c. Stroke volume is high
    d. Atrial "v" wave is low

CASE NO. 23: OBSTRUCTIVE CARDIOMYOPATHY

AB, a twenty-two-year-old college student, is referred to a cardiologist for evaluation of an episode of fainting and a heart murmur.

He describes himself as healthy and very active, a member of his college varsity football team with an intense physical conditioning schedule. He admits that during heavy exercise sessions or at the peak of activity during a game, he sometimes notices mild and transient dizziness. During a recent football game and at the end of running the length of the field, he felt dizzy and fainted for a few seconds. He was taken out of the game and examined. The team physician observed a systolic ejection murmur best heard over the aortic area. This prompted his referral to a cardiologist.

The cardiologist confirms the history, and on physical examination, he reports the following:

- Pulse is 60x', BP is 110/80, normal JVP
- Carotid pulse has a normal to quick upstroke and biispherian.
- Palpable presystolic apical impulse and a strong systolic displacement.
- S1 is normal; S2 is split physiologically at the fourth left space.
- A grade 3/6 ejection systolic murmur that peaks in mid systole is present. No diastolic murmurs noted.
- All peripheral pulses are normal, and the remaining of the physical examination is unremarkable.

ECG shows left ventricular hypertrophy, and chest x-ray is normal.

An echocardiogram is obtained and demonstrated a hypertrophic septum.

DISCUSSION

The age and physical finding could suggest a bicuspid aortic valve. There is, however, a dichotomy between the physical findings and the symptoms. The fainting spell suggests severe stenosis, and the physical findings suggest a milder degree of obstruction. A new diagnosis, obstructive cardiomyopathy, should be considered.

What is the pathophysiology of obstructive cardiomyopathy?

Obstructive cardiomyopathy is caused by localized myocardial hypertrophy, often in the ventricular septum. That results in the following

- A pressure gradient can be recorded inside the ventricular chamber.
- Changes in contractility. Preload, or afterload changes will affect the pressure gradient and the murmur.
- The increase in pressure gradient resulting from changes in contractility may lead to syncope, resulting from an abrupt drop in blood pressure.
- Increases in ventricular volume increase contractility and can therefore increase the pressure gradient. A good example, as shown in the figure below, is a premature ventricular beat. The long postextrasystolic period increases ventricular volume, and as a result, contractility increases and so does the gradient.

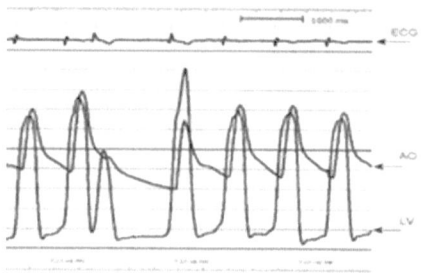

- Myocardial O_2 demand increases, and symptoms of coronary insufficiency may develop.
- Activation of the ventricle always starts from apex to base; therefore, at the start of systole, the area of the septum that will cause the obstruction has yet to activate and obstruction may not exist and no gradient recorded. As activation proceeds, the obstructive area of the septum will contract, exacerbating the obstruction. This will explain the characteristics of arterial pulse, to be discussed below.
- Electrical instability of the myocardium caused by the resulting ischemia can lead to sudden death.
- Diastolic heart failure may develop resulting from the decreased compliance secondary to the hypertrophy.

All of the above will explain the physical findings.

- The carotid pulse will have "bispherians" characteristics. The initial upstroke reflects normal flow before the obstruction develops. Subsequently, a decrease in flow will happen after the obstruction develops.
- The pressure gradient will change as a result of a number of factors and maneuvers, such as the following:
    - Hypovolemia
    - Exercise
    - Tachycardia
    - Postextrasystolic period

- Standing
- Valsalva
- Administration of isoproterenol, nitroglycerin, and amyl nitrate.

* The obstruction will create turbulence in the flow, generating an ejection systolic murmur.

* A murmur of mitral regurgitation is common, caused by abnormalities in the anterior leaflet caused by the recurring impact of the septum on the leaflet with each systole.

* Since the leaflets of the aortic valve are not affected, no ejection click and no changes in S2 will be noted.

* An S4 is frequent as a result of the decreased compliance.

The long-term outcome for people with hypertrophic cardiomyopathy is generally excellent, especially in those diagnosed later in life. With modern treatments, mortality is very low. The vast majority of patients will have normal life expectancy without incurring any significant limiting symptoms or adverse complications. The risk of sudden death after extreme exercise remains a possibility.

TREATMENT

Treatment options are diverse and could include the following:

- Drugs that decrease myocardial contractility, such as beta-blockers

- Pacemakers to alter the sequence of activation of the left ventricle
- Surgical resection of the septum
- Alcohol injection to the septum to cause reduction in the obstructing muscle mass

CASE 23 QUESTIONS

1. A twenty-two-year-old diagnosed with obstructive cardiomyopathy is involved in an auto accident and is bleeding profusely when he arrives to the ED. He is hypovolemic. The impact of the acute hypovolemia on his pressure gradient will

    a. Have no effect
    b. Decrease
    c. Increase
    d. Influence other factors

2. In a patient with obstructive cardiomyopathy, increasing afterload will

    a. Not affect the gradient
    b. Decrease the gradient
    c. Increase the gradient
    d. Decrease the murmur

3. Administration of a drug that decreases afterload will

    a. Increase the gradient
    b. Not affect the gradient
    c. Decrease the intensity of the murmur
    d. Not alter ventricular volume

4. In a patient with obstructive cardiomyopathy, the pressure volume curve will show

    a. Increased stroke volume
    b. Increased end-systolic volume
    c. Increased end-diastolic pressure
    d. Decreased peak systolic pressure

5. A twenty-two-year-old college athlete faints during a demanding practice. The diagnosis of obstructive cardiomyopathy had been made by the echocardiography. The most likely explanation for the fainting includes

   a. CNS disease
   b. Psychosomatic disorder
   c. Increased gradient
   d. Hypervolemia

PERICARDIAL DISEASE

CASE NO. 24: CARDIAC TAMPONADE

AR, a sixty-eight-year-old female, was brought to the ED by her family because of very progressive fatigue and severe shortness of breath that were limiting all activities of daily life and her ability to walk inside the house. These symptoms had started few days before but, in the last few hours, had exacerbated, and now she was unable to perform routine daily activities inside the house.

She explained that she had a right mastectomy five years ago and had recovered well. In a recent follow-up visit, the oncologist noted some metastatic changes in her ribs and vertebra, and she started on a course of radiation therapy plus hormones.

On arrival to the hospital, she appeared very ill, pale and cyanotic. BP was 86 systolic, pulse 100 x', and respiration 20x'.

Physical examination revealed the following:

- Distended jugular veins and weak arterial pulses.
- Chest revealed scar of a right mastectomy.
- Cardiac examination showed that apical impulse was not palpable, and heart sounds were distant.
- A three-component pericardial friction rub was heard.
- BP was 60/46 during inspiration and 80/60 during expiration
- Moderate pitting edema was present in both lower extremities.

A chest x-ray obtained in the ED showed increased cardiac silhouette compatible with a large pericardial effusion.

The ECG is also very helpful in the diagnosis and often shows decrease in QRS amplitude and electrical alternans, manifested by alternating amplitude or morphology of the QRS complex.

Patient was admitted and immediately underwent a procedure with prompt relief of her shortness of breath and normalization of blood pressure.

DISCUSSION

The history of breast cancer, the symptoms, the large cardiac silhouette compatible with a large pericardial effusion, the QRS alternans in the electrocardiogram, the distended neck veins, and the pulsus paradoxus are all indicative of cardiac tamponade, probably secondary to pericardial metastasis.

What is the pathophysiology of cardiac tamponade?

- Pericardial compliance is altered. The pericardium is a fibrous sack with very limited distensibility. When fluid begins to accumulate, pericardial compliance will determine the pressure/volume relationship of the pericardial sac, and this will influence cardiac function.
    - If the accumulation is rapid, as it happens with penetrating trauma or cardiac rupture, a limited amount of fluid will result in rapid increase in pericardial pressure (limited compliance).
    - If the accumulation occurs slowly, the pericardial sac has the opportunity to stretch, and large volumes can accumulate

with little changes in intrapericardial pressure (increased compliance).

- Intrapericardial pressure may reach a certain level that will interfere with diastolic filling of the ventricle—a good example of limitation in preload.

- As a result, end diastolic ventricular volume will decrease and stroke volume will be lower.

- A compensatory response to maintain cardiac output is an increase in heart rate.

- The elevated pericardial pressure isolates the heart from the intrathoracic pressure changes during the respiratory cycle. Under normal circumstances, inspiration lowers intrathoracic pressure, and this is transmitted to the intraardiac pressures that fluctuate during breathing

- In the presence of cardiac tamponade, respiratory variations will not be detectable in the cardiac chambers. Pressures will increase (instead of decreasing during inspiration), reflecting the inspiratory increase in flow and volume during inspiration in all right-sided chambers.

- The increase in RV volume will result in a displacement of the ventricular septum inward toward the left ventricle, one of the main factors in explaining the physiology of pulsus paradoxus. This phenomenon is known as interdependence.

- Another factor in the physiology of cardiac tamponade and pulsus paradoxus is the impact of an elevated intrapericardial pressure on the atrial pressures. The elevation of intrapericardial pressure results in elevation in the right and left atrial pressure. The elevation of the right atrial pressure causes high venous pressure leading to peripheral edema, and the left atrial pressure leads to pulmonary congestion.

- Also, resulting from the elevation of pericardial pressure is that inflow into the left atria will decrease during inspiration because the pulmonary veins respond to changes in intrathoracic pressure while the left atria is isolated from this drop. This creates a negative gradient between the left atria and the pulmonary vein that limits inspiratory filling of the left side.

What are the clinical manifestations of elevated pericardial pressure?

All of the above hemodynamic changes will cause the common symptoms and findings in cardiac tamponade:

- Fatigue (low cardiac output)
- Shortness of breath (elevated capillary pressure)
- Elevated venous pressure (restricted inflow)
- Pulsus paradoxicus (see above)
- Hypotension (decreased cardiac output)
- Tachycardia (compensatory reflex)
- Peripheral cyanosis (low cardiac output)
- Peripheral edema (high right atrial pressure)
- Hepatomegaly (high right atrial pressure)

Electrocardiographic presence of electrical alternans, as shown in this case, is often seen in cardiac tamponade. Electrical alternans is due to alternation in the position of the heart with relation to recording electrodes. Electrical alternans is seen in only 5–10% of patients with cardiac tamponade.

The following are some of the causes of acute pericardial tamponade:

- Malignant diseases—30–60% of cases
- Uremia—10–15% of cases
- Idiopathic pericarditis—5–15%
- Infectious diseases—5–10%
  - HIV
  - Viral (very rare)
- Anticoagulation—5–10%
- Dissecting aneurysm
- Acute MI with myocardial rupture
- Connective tissue diseases—2–6%
- Dressler or postpericardiotomy syndrome—1–2%
- Trauma
  - Blunt
  - Penetrating

TREATMENT

THE EMERGENCY MEDICAL TREATMENT

- Increase preload to maintain blood pressure and cardiac output. Intravenous administration of fluid at a rapid rate can elevate atrial pressure and consequently increase cardiac output. This is only supportive therapy.
- Pericardiocentesis should be performed as an emergency procedure and can rapidly normalize the hemodynamic situation, restore

blood pressure, remove pulsus paradoxus, and improve cardiac output.

SURGICAL TREATMENT

If the underlying process has a likelihood of fluid reaccumulation, a pericardial window should be performed, allowing drainage of pericardial fluid into the pleural cavity.

The following are some of the indications for a pericardial window:

- Symptomatic pericardial effusions
- Pathological/cytologic diagnosis of pericardial effusion
- Hemodynamically stable patients with an undiagnosed large pericardial effusion
- Effusions that reaccumulate after aspiration
- Drainage of a purulent pericardial effusion
- Early fungal or tuberculous pericarditis in which resection of the pericardium is required to prevent future pericardial constriction
- Delayed hemopericardium or effusions after cardiac surgery

The long-term prognosis of cardiac tamponade is related to the disease causing it.

CASE 24 QUESTIONS

1. Pericardial compliance

    a. Determines the filling of cardiac chambers
    b. Does not determine the onset of tamponade
    c. Is more limited in chronic than in acute effusion
    d. Does not influence preload

2. Pulsus paradoxus is seen in cardiac tamponade. It happens because of

    a. Myocardial failure
    b. Respiratory rate
    c. Septal movement
    d. Atrial wall collapse

3. Cardiac tamponade will develop when

    a. Cardiac output drops
    b. Respiratory rate is half of cardiac rate
    c. Pericardial pressure exceeds cardiac filling pressure
    d. Right atrial pressure exceeds left atrial pressure

4. In cardiac tamponade

    a. Afterload is affected
    b. Venous return is increased
    c. Preload decreases
    d. Contractility is impaired

5. When cardiac tamponade develops

    a. Inspiration lowers ventricular systolic pressure
    b. Intracardiac pressure follows changes in intrathoracic pressure

c. Intracardiac pressure reflects flow more than pressure changes
d. Venous return ceases to change with inspiration

6. Emergency management of cardiac tamponade needs

    a. Decreased peripheral vascular resistance
    b. Decreased afterload
    c. Decreased preload
    d. Increased preload

CASE NO. 25. CONSTRICTIVE PERICARDITIS

JR is a sixty-seven-year-old physician who presents for a cardiac evaluation, having noted over the last eight months increasing peripheral edema. He reports no dyspnea or chest pain under any circumstances. He has remained active, walking at least a mile a day and without symptoms.

Physical examination reveals

- moderate distension of jugular veins,
- a 16 mm Hg inspiratory drop in systolic blood pressure,
- an S3 of medium frequency, and
- peripheral edema, moderate.

Characteristically, a chest CT, in this case, shows a thick layer of calcification in the pericardium.

Further history was obtained, and the patient reported that at age thirty, he had several bouts of viral pericarditis with all the characteristic findings, including a large pericardial effusion.

He has remained asymptomatic for all these decades until recently when he noted the onset of symptoms.

DISCUSSION

The history of acute pericarditis several decades before, leading to the current presentation, strongly suggests the early stages of constrictive pericarditis, which is also strongly suggested by the heavy collection of calcium in the pericardial sac.

Constrictive pericarditis occurs when a thickened, fibrotic, or calcified pericardium impedes normal diastolic filling of the heart. This usually involves the parietal pericardium, although it can also involve the visceral pericardium.

The history of the disease, as demonstrated in this case, starts with acute and subacute forms of pericarditis depositing fibrin or a pericardial effusion that may have happened years or decades before.

Also, the physical findings are compatible with the diagnosis. Pericardial knock is a classical finding occurring at the end of rapid ventricular filling (timing like S3), distended jugular veins, and peripheral edema that resulted from the elevated right atrial pressure.

In this case, the layer of calcium in the pericardial sac makes the diagnosis easy. The differential diagnosis includes restrictive cardiomyopathy. Any inflammation of the pericardium, if associated with long-term survival, can lead to constrictive pericarditis. The most common causes of pericarditis that can lead to constriction are as follows:

- Virus
- Bacteria
    - Tuberculosis
- Uremia
- Neoplasia
- Radiation
- Trauma
- Cardiac surgery
- Idiopathic

Incidence of constrictive pericarditis is 0.76 cases per 1,000 person-years after acute idiopathic/viral pericarditis, 31.7 cases for 1,000 person-years for acute tuberculous pericarditis and 52.7 cases per 1,000 person-years for purulent pericarditis.

What is the pathophysiology of constrictive pericarditis?

In constrictive pericarditis, the parietal and visceral pericardial linings become inflamed, thickened, and fused, obliterating the potential space between. As a result the following hemodynamic changes can happen:

- The ventricles lose distensibility.
- Limited venous return to the heart .
- Filling of the ventricles is reduced.
- Preload of the ventricles is decreased.
- End-diastolic volume is decreased.
- Right and left end-diastolic pressures are increased
- Cardiac output and stroke volume are decreased.
- **Filling pressures of the heart tend to become equal in both the ventricles and the atria.**
- The myocardium, unless infiltrated by calcium (seen very late in the disease), retains normal contractility, and systolic function remains unaffected.
- During the development of the constriction, right and left ventricular diastolic pressure are increased.
- A small increase in volume results in a considerable increase in end-diastolic pressure.

Symptoms consistent with congestive heart failure (CHF), especially right-sided heart failure, develop as a result of the inability of the heart to fill properly. Over time, cardiac output gradually becomes inadequate.

The clinical symptoms and classic hemodynamic findings of constrictive pericarditis can be explained by the early rapid diastolic filling and elevation, with eventual equalization of the diastolic pressures in all the cardiac chambers. This restricts late diastolic filling, leading to venous engorgement and decreased cardiac output, all secondary to a confined pericardium.

TREATMENT

Treatment is surgical, necessitating the careful dissection of the calcified pericardium. Supportive therapy to include diuretics must be used with care since they can lower cardiac output and arterial pressure.

Results are generally better if the pericardiectomy is performed earlier in the clinical course, when less calcification is present and when the chance of abnormal fibrotic myocardium is less of an issue.

Surgical mortality ranges from 5–15%, but survival is associated with a functional return to NYHA class I or II.

CASE 25 QUESTIONS

1. In patients with constrictive pericarditis, end-systolic volume is

    a. Normal
    b. Increased
    c. Decreased

2. A common hemodynamic finding in constrictive pericarditis is

    a. Increased end-diastolic volume
    b. Equalization of pressures in all chambers
    c. Increased end-systolic volume
    d. Increased stroke volume

3. The differential diagnosis of constrictive pericarditis include

    a. Acute myocarditis
    b. Dilated cardiomyopathy
    c. Cardiomyopathy
    d. Cardiac amyloidosis

4. In patients with constrictive pericarditis

    a. End-diastolic volume increases
    b. Stroke volume increases
    c. End-systolic volume decreases
    d. Afterload increases

5. Patients with acute MI develop constrictive pericarditis

    a. Very rarely
    b. Often

6. The silent interval between acute and constrictive pericarditis is

    a. Days
    b. Months
    c. Years

CARDIAC ARRHYTHMIAS

CASE NO. 26: COMPLETE HEART BLOCK

TT, a seventy-five-year-old retired carpenter, has been in his usual state of good health, is free of any cardiac symptoms, and has able to maintain an exercise routine of walking one mile a day without complaints.

One morning, while on his walking routine, he begins to feel dizzy and, shortly after, faints, losing consciousness for a few seconds. His walking companion realizes what is happening and, with his cell phone, calls 911. An ambulance arrives and transports him to a local hospital. In route to the hospital, they obtain an EG that is transmitted to the ED.

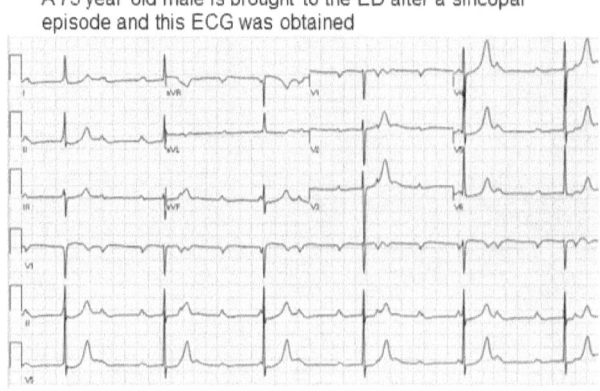

A 75 year old male is brought to the ED after a sincopal episode and this ECG was obtained

Fig. 25.1. The rhythm strip is shown below with an atrial rate of 90 per minute and a ventricular rate of 30 per minute. There is no relationship between P and QRS complexes, and the QRS is wide (0.12 seconds). Diagnosis: complete AV block

Upon arrival to the hospital, the ECG is repeated, showing the same findings of a complete AV block with an idioventricular rhythm.

Patient is admitted to the hospital, a temporary pacemaker is inserted, and twenty-four hours later, a permanent pacemaker is installed.

DISCUSSION

This case illustrates the common presentation of a complete heart block.

The rhythm strip presented above shows P waves and QRS complexes having no temporal relationship.

THE CONDUCTION SYSTEM

Before we address the various potential anatomical location of a heart block, a brief review of the conduction system of the heart is necessary

SINOATRIAL NODE

The SA node is located at the junction of the anteromedial aspect of the superior vena cava (SVC) and the right atrium (RA). The blood supply is from the sinus node branches of the right coronary artery in 55–60% of hearts or the left circumflex artery in 40–45% of hearts.

The SA node is densely innervated with adrenergic and cholinergic nerve terminals and generates impulses slightly faster than any other area. The pacemaker potential creates 60 to 110 action potentials per minute, thus overdriving all other areas with automaticity, a phenomenon named overdrive suppression.

As the electrical activity is spreading throughout the atria, the impulse travels from the SA node to the AV node via three specialized pathways, known as anterior, middle, and posterior internodal pathway.

ATRIOVENTRICULAR NODE

The **atrioventricular node** is located in the posteroinferior region of the interatrial septum near the opening of the coronary sinus. The blood supply of the AV node is via the AV nodal artery that, in about 80–90% of hearts, is a branch of the right coronary artery.

The specific properties and function of the AV node are as follows:

- It delays impulse transmission to the ventricles by approximately 0.12 seconds. This delay is important because it insures that the atria have filled the ventricles before the ventricles contract.

- Its longer refractory period protects the ventricles from a very fast rate that is deleterious to cardiac function.

- It can conduct impulses in both directions (forward and retrograde), important in the physiology of some rhythm disturbances.

- Unique to the AV node is **decremental conduction**, indicating that the faster the node is stimulated, the longer it will take to conduct. This is the property of the AV node that prevents rapid conduction to the ventricle in case of rapid atrial rhythms.

- Its automaticity is 40–60 times per minute, allowing to become a backup pacemaker in case of SA node failure.

AV conduction during normal cardiac rhythm occurs through two different pathways (this is an important concept understanding reentry arrhythmias):

- ○ The first pathway has a slow conduction velocity but shorter refractory period.
- ○ The second pathway has a faster conduction velocity but longer refractory period.

BUNDLE OF HIS

The **bundle of His** connects with the distal part of the AV node and eventually penetrates the membranous septum.

Branches from the anterior and posterior descending coronary arteries supply the upper muscular interventricular septum, which makes the conduction system protected from the acute ischemic damages.

BUNDLE BRANCHES

Bundle branches originate below the membranous septum.

- ○ The left bundle branch moves to the septum beneath the noncoronary aortic cusp.
- ○ The left bundle divides into two fascicles:
  - The anterior fascicle, long and thin, is directed toward the lateral wall of the left ventricle.

- - The posterior fascicle is directed toward the inferior and posterior wall of the left ventricle.
  - ○ The anatomy of the left bundle branch system may be variable and not conform to the concept of a bifascicular division. However, for clinical purposes and electrocardiography, the concept of a trifascicular system with two segments originating from the left bundle remains useful.
  - ○ The right bundle branch continues as an unbranched extension of the AV bundle down the right side of the interventricular septum to the apex of the right ventricle and base of the anterior papillary muscle.

TERMINAL PURKINJE FIBERS

Terminal Purkinje fibers connect with the ends of the bundle branches to form interweaving networks on the endocardial surface of both ventricles, which transmit the cardiac impulse almost simultaneously to the entire right and left ventricular endocardium.

An important concept that must be emphasized is the proximity of the conduction system to the aortic and mitral rings. Calcification of the rings, a common issue with aging, is likely to allow for fibrous and calcium deposits in the conduction system leading to heart block, bundle branch block, or any other abnormality in impulse conduction.

In patients with complete heart block, where is the block anatomically located?

The most common cause of complete heart block is fibrosis of the conduction system occurring in ether the distal portion of the common bundle or the right bundle branch and both segments of the left (trifascicular block). This is the common cause in heart block in elderly populations, with a higher prevalence of males over women

The block could also be located in the AV node or caused by fibrosis or tumors in the AV node. In this case, the dominant rhythm originates in the AV junction, has a faster rate than an idioventricular rhythm (40–50 x'), and can slightly increase rate through the innervation of the AV node.

Bradyarrhythmias may also result from failures in the automaticity of the sinus node as will be demonstrated in a subsequent case.

What are the pathophysiological and hemodynamic changes that happen as a consequence of complete heart block?

The classical findings are as follows:

- Ventricular rate is between 20–30 beats per minute (determined by the anatomical location of the block), with a rate of 50 if block is in the AV node.

- There is no synchronization between P waves and QRS complexes.

- To maintain a good cardiac output, stroke volume is increased through an increase in contractility.

- Increased end-diastolic volume is needed to increase stroke volume. This causes the increase in contractility in the presence of a slow heart rate.

- The increased volume stretches myocardial fibers and increase the rate of contractility.

- There is slight increase in systolic pressure due to increased contractility.

- There are beat-to-beat changes in stroke volume and systolic blood pressure due to the changes in timing relationship between P and QRS. If atrial contraction is timed appropriately with systole (a normal PR interval), the increase in ventricular filling will increase stroke volume and blood pressure.

- Increased end-diastolic volume increases subendocardial pressure.

The physiological changes result in the following physical findings:

- Slow heart rate

- Beat-to-beat changes in arterial pulse amplitude and systolic blood pressure caused by the changing timing of P and QRS that affects the late filling of the ventricles

- Varying intensity of the first heart sound determined by the changing relationship between P and QRS that affect AV valve motion.

- Cannon waves—intermittent visible big "a" waves, visible in the jugular vein, when atrial contraction occurs superimposed with the QRS complex and the tricuspid valve is closed.

- If heart block is untreated, as seen in congenital heart block, left ventricular hypertrophy may develop.

What is the physiological explanation for the loss of consciousness?

The loss of consciousness associated with bradyarrhythmias (commonly known as Stoke-Adams attacks) can be explained as follows:

- In a patient with complete heart block, cardiac output is maintained by a slow idioventricular rhythm at a rate of approximately 30x'. This rate cannot increase substantially to meet with increased physiological demands.
- Any increase in cardiac output must be caused by increased ventricular contractility, already increased as a result of the bradycardia.
- If the patient exercises, it results in peripheral vascular dilatation. It may not be accompanied by increased output through further increase in contractility.
- The result is a drop in blood pressure and loss of consciousness.

What are the common causes of heart block?

- Fibrosis and calcification of the conduction system are the most common causes.
- *It is important to remember that the aortic and mitral rings are anatomically close to the conduction system, and calcification of the valves may easily extend to the conduction system.*
- Repair of congenital lesions (i.e., ventricular septal defects).

- Drugs.
    - Class Ia antiarrhythmics (e.g., quinidine, procainamide, disopyramide)
    - Class Ic antiarrhythmics (e.g., flecainide, encainide, propafenone)
    - Class II antiarrhythmics (beta-blockers)
    - Class III antiarrhythmics (e.g., amiodarone, sotalol, dofetilide, ibutilide)
    - Class IV antiarrhythmics (calcium channel blockers)
    - Digoxin or other cardiac glycosides

Much less frequent causes are as follows

- Mitral or aortic valve repair
- Ablation procedures
- Tumor infiltration
- Rheumatic diseases—ankylosing spondylitis, Reiter syndrome, relapsing polychondritis, rheumatoid arthritis, scleroderma
- Infiltrative processes—amyloidosis, sarcoidosis, tumors, Hodgkin disease, multiple myeloma
- Neuromuscular disorders—Becker muscular dystrophy, myotonic muscular dystrophy
- Myocardial infarction
- Metabolic causes—hypoxia, hyperkalemia, hypothyroidism
- Toxins—mad honey (grayanotoxin)

TREATMENT

Treatment of heart block demands implantation of a pacemaker. Until a permanent pacemaker is inserted, a temporary pacemaker or an external pacemaker can be used.

The type of permanent pacemaker to be used varies, but most commonly it is a demand pacemaker, able to recognize underlying rhythm. Modern pacemakers have a number of features that maximize their clinical advantage, such atrioventricular synchronized pacemakers, capable of stimulating both chamber with a predetermined PR interval.

There is no long-term medical treatment for heart block. In emergencies, drugs that increase ventricular automaticity, such as isoproterenol, or drugs that improve AV conduction offer transient relief.

CASE 26 QUESTIONS

1. In patients with chronic complete heart block (before insertion of pacemaker)

    a. End-diastolic volume is increased
    b. Pulmonary vascular resistance increases
    c. Stroke volume decreases
    d. Contractility decreases

2. The most common site of a complete heart block is

    a. Sinoatrial junction
    b. AV node
    c. Ventricular conduction system
    d. Purkinje system

3. In patients with complete heart block

    a. Systolic blood pressure is likely to increase
    b. Contractility decreases
    c. Stroke volume decreases
    d. Peripheral vascular resistance decreases

4. One of the following can cause heart block

    a. Aortic stenosis
    b. Mitral stenosis
    c. Ventricular aneurysm repair
    d. Pericardial window

5. Congenital heart block can

    a. Cause aortic regurgitation
    b. Cause left ventricular hypertrophy
    c. Cause mitral regurgitation
    d. Cause mitral stenosis

CASE NO. 27: BRADYARRHYTHMIAS—SICK SINUS SYNDROME

JJ, an eighty-two-year-old lady, presents complaining of frequent episodes of dizziness without any fainting episodes. A comprehensive examination fails to show any neurological abnormalities to explain the symptoms. The only finding reported was an intermittent slow heart rate and long pauses up to five seconds.

She is referred for a cardiological evaluation. A Holter monitor was obtained that shows multiple episodes of escape junctional rhythm and no visible atrial activity.

DISCUSSION

Sick sinus syndrome is a disorder characterized by a dysfunctional sinus node. It is often idiopathic and a result of degenerative fibrosis. It can also be caused by

- amyloidosis,
- connective tissue disease,
- Chagas disease,
- hemochromatosis,
- hypertensive heart disease,
- cardiomyopathies, and
- drugs such as digitalis, calcium channel blockers, β-blockers, sympatholytic agents, and several antiarrhythmic drugs.

What is the electrophysiology of sick sinus syndrome?

There are several potential mechanisms for this disorder:

- The sinus node may not fire at all (SA arrest).
- An impulse cannot activate the atria because of SA block (block between the SA node and the atrial myocardium).
- The SA node may discharge, but if the impulse is blocked, the atrium will not be depolarized, and consequently, P waves will not be present.

This syndrome is often accompanied by disease or depression of the junctional tissue.

The electrocardiographic findings include

- sinus bradycardia,
- sinus arrest or SA block,
- SA arrest with escape atrial or junctional rhythms,
- SA arrest with failure of subsidiary pacemaker resulting in asystole,
- bradycardia alternating with tachycardia, and
- chronic atrial fibrillation with failure of sinus rhythm to return after cardioversion.

The most common symptoms include fainting, dizziness, worsening heart failure, palpitations, and multiple rhythm disorders.

Many patients with SSS may have more than one rhythm abnormality. Bradycardia-tachycardia is more common in the elderly with SSS, and atrial fibrillation is the most common arrhythmia. Paroxysmal supraventricular tachycardia, atrial flutter, and atrial tachycardia. It is important to determine whether the AF is associated with SSS. Treating AF with cardioversion or medication but without a supporting pacemaker can result in prolonged periods of asystole. In the absence of bradycardia resulting from drug therapy (i.e., digitalis, β-blockers), an abnormal sinus node physiology should be considered.

TREATMENT

Treatment usually requires a pacemaker.

It is important to remember that drugs that depress automaticity and conduction may cause advanced sinus bradycardia. Temporary discontinuation of the drug may eliminate sick sinus syndrome.

CASE 27 QUESTIONS

1. Potential causes of sick sinus syndrome include

    a. Amyloidosis
    b. Idiopathic
    c. Chagas disease
    d. All of the above
    e. None of the above

2. Sinus recovery time is

    a. The P-P interval
    b. P-P interval at fast rates
    c. When time for a sinus P wave appears after a period of tachycardia or atrial pacing
    d. Short recovery time indicates disease of the sinus node
    e. All of the above

3. Arrhythmias observed with sick sinus rhythm include

    a. Atrial fibrillation
    b. Supraventricular tachycardia
    c. Alternating supraventricular tachycardia and sinus bradycardia
    d. All of the above
    e. None of the above

4. Antiarrhytmic drugs can cause sick sinus rhythm

    a. True
    b. False

CASE NO. 28: WENCKEBACH PHENOMENA

AA, an eighty-two-year-old male with a longstanding history of hypertension and angina pectoris, had been treated with a beta-blocker for some time. In the last few weeks, the patient noted a slight increase on the frequency of his mild anginal episodes and proceeded on his own, without consulting his physician, to double the dose of his beta-blocker.

He went to his physician office for a regular follow-up visit. The physician took the patient's pulse and noted an irregularity. They proceeded to take a rhythm strip (shown below). Based on the findings, the patient was advised to return to the old dose and to return in a week for a follow-up visit.

2nd degree heart block type one

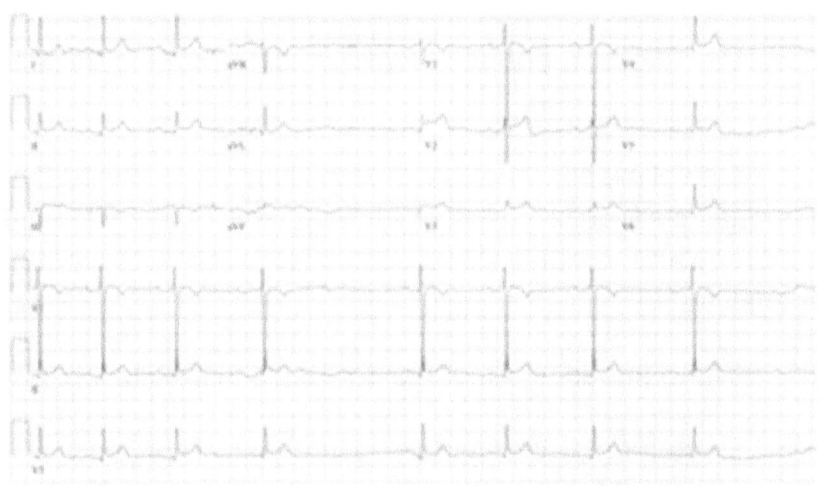

Fig. 28.1. The rhythm strip shows normal sinus rhythm and a progressive prolongation of the PR that culminates in a nonconducted P wave. The QRS complex has normal duration and morphology.

DISCUSSION

The criteria for the diagnosis of a second-degree heart block, type 1, or Wenckebach phenomena include the following:

- Progressive prolongation of the PR interval on consecutive beats followed by a nonconducted P wave.

- Secondary criteria include the following:

    ◦ The first conducted P wave after the block will have the shortest PR interval.

    ◦ The **prolongation** of PR is the longest in the second conducted beat.

    ◦ **Increment** in subsequent PR intervals is progressively shorter.

    ◦ The **RR interval** is progressively shorter.

Wenckebach phenomena is almost always a disease of the AV node.

One of the baseline assumptions when determining if an individual has Mobitz 1 heart block is that the atrial rhythm has to be regular and at least two conducted beats are available for analysis.

There are some fundamental points in Mobitz 1 block:

- Decremental conduction is present. This topic was addressed in a previous case and is a property of the AV node.

- The atrial rate at which Mobitz 1 develops is indicative of the refractory period of the AV node.

- Mobitz 1 is almost always a benign condition for which no emergency treatment is needed. In symptomatic cases, intravenous atropine or isoproterenol may transiently improve conduction, and a pacemaker may be indicated.

Causes of Mobitz 1 block are as follows:

- Vagal stimulated AV block can also be associated with ECG evidence of sinus slowing.

High vagal tone can occur in young patients or athletes at rest and can be observed in 2–10% of long-distance runners. A vagally mediated AV block improves with exercise and may occur more commonly during sleep, when parasympathetic tone dominates.

- Cardioactive drugs are an important cause of AV block. They may exert negative effect on the conductivity of the AVN directly or through the autonomic nervous system or both. The following are the drugs that commonly cause Wenkebach phenomena:
    - Digoxin
    - Beta-blockers
    - Calcium channel blockers

Other potential reasons for Mobitz 1 are the following:

- Acute myocardial infarction.
- Endocarditis causing AV nodal abscesses.
- Lyme disease.
- Acute rheumatic fever.
- Infiltrative diseases such as amyloidosis, hemochromatosis, and sarcoidosis.
- Infiltrative malignancies such as Hodgkin lymphoma and other lymphomas.

- ○ Hyperkalemia, hypermagnesemia.
- ○ Myxedema.
- ○ Collagen vascular diseases.
- ○ Cardiac tumors.
- ○ Trauma.
    a. Catheter related.
    b. Ethanol septal reduction used for the treatment of obstructive. hypertrophic cardiomyopathy.
    c. Correction of congenital heart diseases (i.e., ASD, VSD).
    d. Valvular heart disease.
    e. Catheter ablation procedures.
- ○ Genetic—AV block may be autosomal dominant. Mutations in the *N5A* gene have been linked to familial AV block.

TREATMENT

Treatment is a function of the cause of block.

Temporary discontinuation of drugs capable of prolonging AV node refractory period usually restores normal conduction.

Treatment of the underlying cause may restore normal conduction. A pacemaker may be indicated in some patients depending on symptoms.

CASE 28 QUESTIONS

1. Wenckebach phenomena is associated with

    a. Increased automaticity
    b. Decreased automaticity
    c. Longer AV node refractory period
    d. Shortened AV node refractory period

2. Mobitz 1 is often a physiologic phenomenon related to

    a. Increased automaticity
    b. Parasympathetic stimulation
    c. Sympathetic stimulation
    d. Decreased refractory period

3. In Mobitz 1

    a. QRS is always normal
    b. Shortest PR is first conducted after the block
    c. RR interval remains constant
    d. Last PR interval is the shortest

4. In Mobitz 1

    a. AV node refractory period is short
    b. AV node refractory period is prolonged
    c. Automaticity is increased
    d. Contractility is decreased

CASE NO. 29: MOBITZ 2

RP is a seventy-eight-year-old male who presents to the ED after a brief syncopal episode. His past neurological history is negative, and his cardiovascular history reports that he had an abnormal ECG with bundle branch block for several years. He denies any previous dizziness or fainting spells.

A rhythm strip is obtained on admission and is shown below, demonstrating Mobitz 2 block.

2nd degree heart block Mobitz 2 type

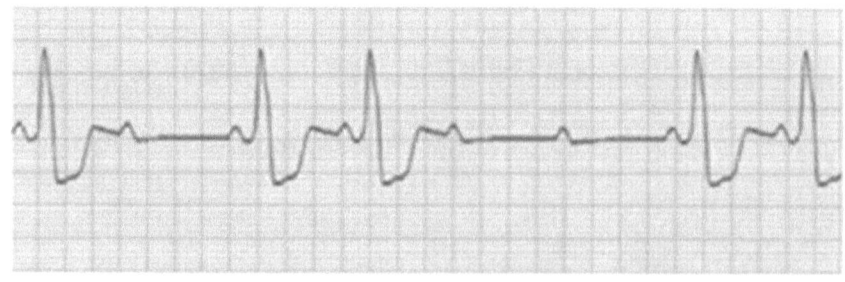

Fig. 29.1.

The patient is admitted, and a permanent pacemaker is inserted the next day.

DISCUSSION

Type 2 second-degree AV block, also known as Mobitz 2, almost always results from disease of the distal conduction system.

The electrocardiographic features are as follows:

- Intermittently nonconducted P waves not preceded by PR prolongation and not followed by PR shortening

- Prolongation of QRS denoting a ventricular conduction defect

- Constant RR interval for all conducted beats

Mobitz type 2 AV block may progress rapidly to complete heart block, in which no escape rhythm may emerge or may be a very slow ventricular rate, inadequate for hemodynamic support. The person may experience a Stokes-Adams attack (loss of consciousness caused by a bradyarrhythmia), cardiac arrest, or sudden cardiac death. The definitive treatment is an implanted permanent pacemaker.

The impairment of conduction is almost always below the AV node in the distal conduction system at or below the His bundle.

In the case of a 2:1 block, there are not enough cycles to demonstrate that the PR is prolonging (Mobitz 1) or is constant (Mobitz 2). It is therefore impossible to differentiate type 1 from type 2 Mobitz block, based solely on the P-QRS ratio. The proper terminology would be advanced second-degree A-V block.

The ability to make this differentiation is of practical and prognostic significance. In the absence of intracavitary ECG recordings and electrophysiological studies, how can we predict the type? Some clues are as follows:

- A lengthened PR interval with a normal QRS duration is most likely indicative of a type 1 with the disease in the AV node.

- A normal PR interval with a widened QRS is most likely indicative of a type 2 with the disease in the distal conduction system. In such cases, a permanent pacemaker insertion is the treatment of choice since the rhythm is unpredictable and the risk of asystole high.

TRIFASCICULAR BLOCK

We will conclude this case with a brief review of concepts important in the understanding of heart block and conduction defects.

- The conducting system of the heart consists specialized cells that can initiate impulses and conduct them rapidly through the heart.

- The bundle branches begin immediately below the membranous septum.

- The left bundle branch goes onto the septum beneath the noncoronary aortic cusp.

- Left bundle branch system may be variable in morphology. In many cases it subdivides into the following:

    ○ *Left anterior division.* Long and thin, it distributes to the anterolateral wall of the left ventricle. Fibrosis, commonly seen with many cases of left ventricular hypertrophy, causes marked left axis deviation (minus thirty degrees or higher) and is also called left anterior fascicular block.

- ○ *Left posterior division.* Thick and short, it distributes to the interoposterior wall of the left ventricle. Because of its length and thickness, posterior hemiblock is a rare clinical finding. Left posterior fascicular block results in right axis deviation.

- ○ The anatomy of the conduction system may be variable. It may not always conform to bifascicular division, although the concept is important for a better understanding of conduction defects.

* The right bundle branch continues in the myocardium as an unbranched extension of the AV bundle and travels down the right side of the interventricular septum to the apex of the right ventricle and base of the anterior papillary muscle.

For clinical purposes, the concept of a trifascicular conduction system, consisting of the right bundle branch and the two fascicles of the left bundle (left anterior and left posterior division), is important. This has been demonstrated by a number of authors reporting serial electrocardiograms and by anatomical studies.

CASE 29 QUESTIONS

1. The most common cause of complete heart block is

    a. Congenital lesion in AV node
    b. Tumor infiltration in the conduction system
    c. Fibrosis of the conduction system
    d. Infective endocarditis

2. Bifascicular block always leads to complete AV block

    a. True
    b. False

3. Posterior hemiblock

    a. Causes left axis deviation
    b. Is common
    c. More common with inferior infarction
    d. Is rare

4. Left anterior hemiblock

    a. Is only caused by left ventricular hypertrophy
    b. Is only caused by bi-ventricular hypertrophy
    c. Involves the anterior division of the left bundle
    d. Is caused only by coronary heart disease

5. Complete AV block can be associated with

    a. Genetic anomalies
    b. Endocarditis
    c. Tumors
    d. All of the above

6. In patients with an acute anterior MI, the presence of complete heart block

    a. Is always benign
    b. Commonly associated with a junctional rhythm
    c. Has a poor prognosis
    d. Is always accompanied by cardiogenic shock

CASE NO. 30: SUPRAVENTRICULAR TACHYCARDIA

DD, a forty-six-year-old lady, reports to the ED indicating that she developed a very rapid heart rate. She reports no symptoms other than palpitations and describes that her heart rate is very rapid and regular.

Her past medical and family history is noncontributory. She reports no symptoms suggestive of any cardiovascular disease, and this is the first episode with the characteristics she describes.

On examination, rate is 180 x' and BP is 100/70. Cardiovascular examination reveals no abnormalities and no murmurs.

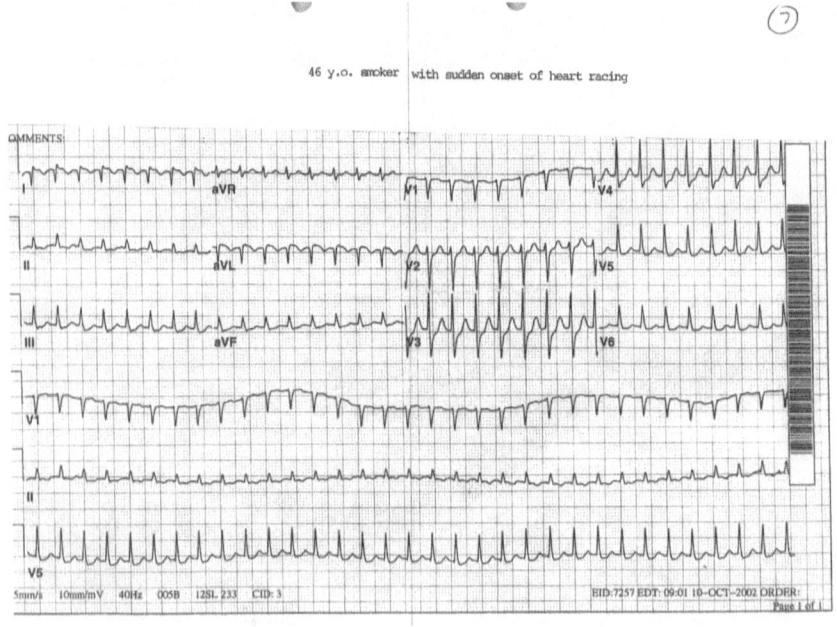

Fig. 30.1. The ECG obtained in the ED is shown above. It reveals a ventricular rate of 175 beats per minute. QRS morphology is normal, and some repolarization changes are seen. The P waves are not easily seen and could be concealed in the ST segment.

The diagnosis of paroxysmal supraventricular tachycardia is made, and the patient is given IV adenosine with prompt return to normal sinus rhythm.

The patient recovered promptly and was discharged to the care of her primary care physician.

DISCUSSION

This is one of the most common arrhythmias seen in the ED.

The characterisics of AV nodal reentry tachycardia (AVNRT) are as follows:

- Diagnosed in 50–60% of patients who present with a regular, narrow QRS tachyarrhythmia.
- The ventricular rate is approximately of 180 per minute.
- Often seen in people older than twenty years.
- Occurs more often in women.
- It is easily treatable and commonly not associated with any underlying heart disease.
- It is a classical example of reentry tachycardia.

ELECTROPHYSIOLOGY OF AV NODAL REENTRY TACHYCARDIA

The basis of AV nodal reentry tachycardia rests on the electrophysiology of the AV node.

The AV node's fundamental function is to protect the ventricles from extremely rapid rates emanating from the atria. To achive this goal, the AV node is equipped with the following:

- A relatively long refractory period, between 300 msec and 400 msec. This will limit the ventricular response from any supraventricular tachycardia to a maximum of 150 to 200 beats per minute.
- Can conduct an electrical impulse antegrade (from atria to ventricle) or retrograde (from ventricle to atria).
- Decremental conduction, discussed earlier, which is part of the mechanism to regulate rate by affecting conduction velocity.
- Rapid rate, faster than the refractory period, will lead to a Wenckebach or Mobitz 1 block.

In 40% of subjects, fibers in the AV node may have two different conduction properties, a critical concept for the understanding of reentry AV nodal tachycardia. These fibers will have different electrophysiological properties.

- One pathway (alpha) is relatively slow conducting, with a short refractory period.
- The second pathway (beta) is a rapid conducting pathway with a long refractory period.

The coexistence of these functionally different pathways is the substrate for AV reentrant tachycardia.

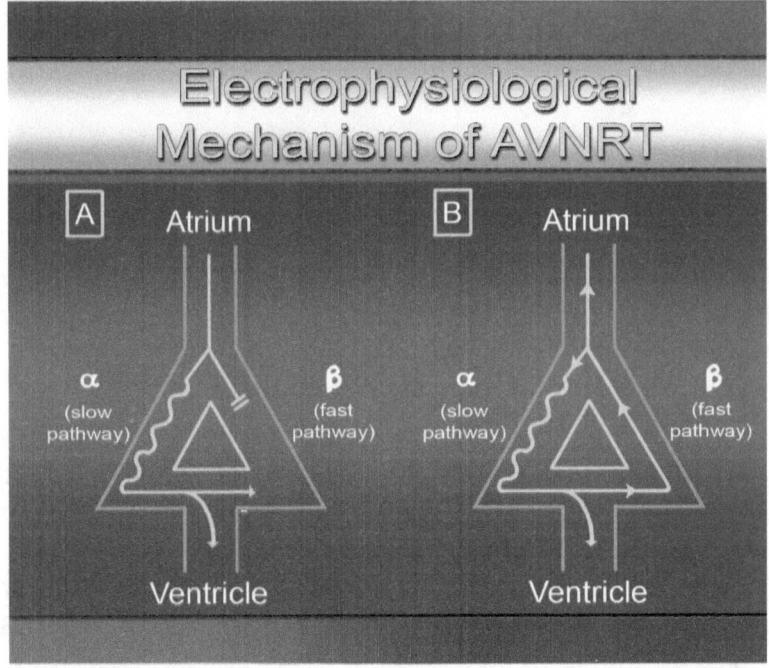

Fig. 29.2. Diagrammatic representation of the reentry phenomena triggered by a premature atrial beat.

As illustrated above, the onset of AVNRT is triggered by a premature atrial impulse that reaches the AV node when the alpha pathway is still refractory from the previous impulse but the beta pathway may be able to conduct. If the slow pathway (alpha) has repolarized by the time the impulse completes retrograde conduction, the impulse can reenter the slow pathway (alpha) and initiate AVNRT. (See the image above.)

The AVNRT does not involve the ventricles as part of the reentry circuit.

Because the impulse typically conducts in an anterograde manner through slow pathway and in a retrograde manner through the fast pathway, the PR interval (antegrade) is longer than the RP interval (retrograde).

In patients with typical AVNRT, the P wave is usually located at the terminal portion of the QRS complex.

TREATMENT

Treatment of AVNRT is based on the electrophysiological concepts explained above: *if antegrade conduction is slowed sufficiently, one beat may fail to conduct, terminating the reentry cycle.*

Vagal stimulation—any maneuver resulting in stimulation of the vagus nerve (i.e., carotid massage, cough, gag reflex) is capable of terminating the AVNRT arrhythmia.

The duration of the resulting arrhythmia is often unpredictable, especially in elderly patients who often have associated sinus node disease. Periods of asystole may be seen when the arrhythmia terminates. The extrasystolic depression of the SA node delays its recovery until it regains control of the atria. During this brief period, electrical instability is increased, and in rare cases, this may be complicated by the onset of ventricular fibrillation.

Drugs that delay AV conduction, such as digoxin, beta-blockers, or calcium channel blockers, can terminate AVNRT. Adenosine is the drug most commonly used in the termination of AVNRT.

CASE 30 QUESTIONS

1. The AV node refractory period

    a. Is constant
    b. Is not influenced by sympathetic stimulation
    c. Will not limit ventricular rate in supraventricular tachycardia
    d. Is affected by carotid stimulation

2. A supraventricular tachycardia

    a. Should have an abnormal QRS complex
    b. The ventricular rate is usually around 300 beats x'
    c. Will always have visible P waves
    d. The P wave will always precede the QRS

3. The ventricular rate in AVNRT

    a. Determined by A-V refractory period
    b. Cannot be faster than 200 x
    c. Is not influenced by sympathetic stimulation
    d. Does not influence QRS duration

4. Carotid sinus stimulation (e.g., carotid massage, coughing, straining, increasing abdominal pressure, or gag reflex)

    a. Always increases atrial rate
    b. Should not be performed in both sides simultaneously
    c. Will always terminate tachycardia
    d. Cannot produce asystole
    e. Does not prolong AV node refractory period

5. The presence of two different conductions in the AV node

    a. Is rare
    b. Always present
    c. Seen in 40% of individuals
    d. Is critical in atrial fibrillation

CASE NO. 31: WOLFF-PARKINSON-WHITE SYNDROME

RP, a thirty-two-year-old male, is applying for a large life insurance policy and visited a primary care physician for a required physical examination. His medical history is negative and has no cardiovascular symptoms.

The BP is 122/80, and physical examination is normal.

The insurance company required an electrocardiogram that is shown below.

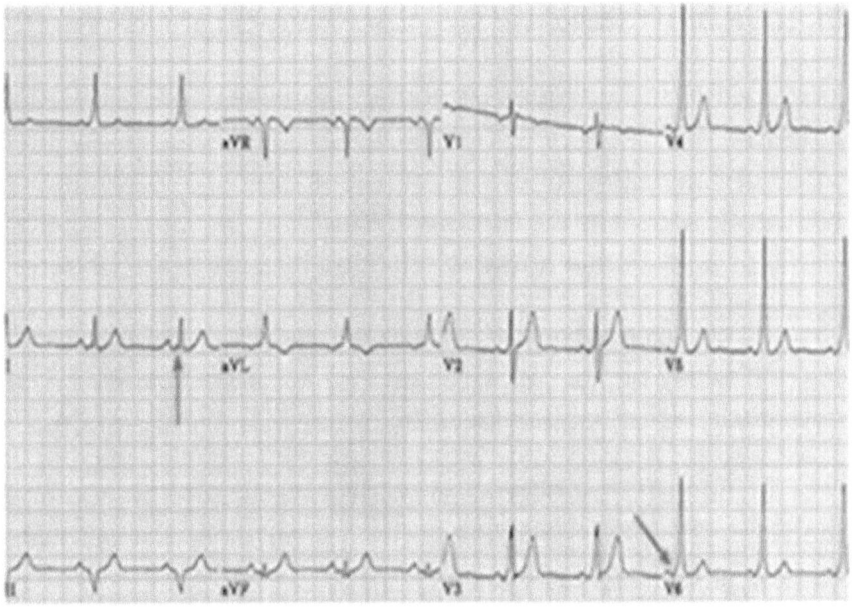

Fig. 31.1. The electrocardiogram shows a normal sinus rhythm, rate is 90, PR is 0.11 se, the QRS duration is 0.11, and there is slurring of the initial component of the QRS compatible with a *delta wave*. The QT interval is normal.

Because of the ECG finding, he is referred to a cardiologist for further evaluation.

DISCUSSION

The ECG criteria to diagnose Wolff-Parkinson-White syndrome include the following:

- Short PR interval (< 0.12 sec)
- PR segment covered by the P wave morphology
- Long QRS (> 0.10 sec)
- Delayed initial QRS forces (slurred) (delta wave)
- Normal QT interval

ELECTROPHYSIOLOGY OF WOLFF-PARKINSON-WHITE

WPW is a congenital anomaly. Impulse conduction from atria to ventricle occurs through an accessory pathway that communicates the atria and the ventricles. This accessory pathway is known as the **bundle of Kent** and may be associated with a protein kinase enzyme encoded by the *PRKAG2* gene.

This accessory pathway conducts electrical activity at a significantly higher velocity than the AV node resulting in a potentially faster ventricular rate if an arrhythmia develops.

The **bundle of Kent** that is present in a small percentage (between 0.1 and 0.3%) of the general population. This pathway may communicate as follows:

- Between the left atrium and the left ventricle, (type A)

- Between the right atrium and the right ventricle, (type B)

The presence of the accessory pathway can result in the bypassing of the AV node and creating the potential for a reentry tachycardia.

In some cases of WPW, antegrade conduction from the atria may occur simultaneously thru both the AV node and the accessory pathway. As a result, the QRS morphology may be a fusion of both possibilities with changes in QRS duration and morphology.

If a subject with WPW develops atrial fibrillation, ventricular rate may be fast ranging from 250 to 300 and determined by the refractory period of the Kent bundle. The explanation is the existing accessory pathway that may have a short refractory period and be able to conduct many of the fibrillatory impulses.

The presence of WPW, if not associated with atrial tachycardia or other arrhythmias, is a relatively benign condition. If complicated by atrial fibrillation, it becomes serious, which has the possibility of sudden death and a shortened life span.

TREATMENT

Patients with WPW but without cardiac arrhythmias do not require specific antiarrhythmic drugs, and the treatment of choice is the destruction of the accessory pathway with ablation.

Treatment of patients with atrial fibrillation and rapid ventricular response may include procainamide to stabilize their heart rate following cardioversion. **Amiodarone** is no longer recommended in this clinical scenario after reports of ventricular fibrillation.

AV node blockers should be avoided in atrial fibrillation and atrial flutter with WPW. These drugs block antegrade impulse conduction through the AV node and may lead to 1:1

atrial to ventricle conduction through the preexcitation pathway, potentially leading to unstable ventricular arrhythmias.

ABLATION

The definitive treatment of WPW is catheter ablation th has a success rate as high as 95%. Recurrence rates are typically less than 5% after a successful ablation.

CASE 31 QUESTIONS

1. WPW is

    a. Acquired
    b. Always associated with well-known genetic anomaly
    c. Always have a benign prognosis
    d. Often accompanies congenital heart lesions

2. The Bundle of Kent

    a. Has a long refractory period
    b. Conducts faster than the A-V node
    c. Is always located in the intra-atrial septum
    d. Can only conduct retrograde

3. Bundle of Kent can

    a. Produce ventricular tachycardia
    b. Conduct an impulse only in an antegrade fashion
    c. Has a refractory period longer than AV node
    d. Conduction velocity is faster than AV node

4. Reentry tachycardia

    a. Always requires an accessory pathway
    b. Requires conduction pathways with different refractory periods
    c. Cannot be cured
    d. Is only caused by WPW

CASE NO. 32: ATRIAL FIBRILLATION

GB is a seventy-eight-year-old retired corporate executive that has been in good health until this event happened. On a Monday morning, when he started a gentle walk, he noted that he was very short of breath and could not walk more than a couple of blocks without having to stop to catch his breath. This was a brand-new event since he had seen his primary care physician a few weeks before and found to be in good general health.

His past medical history was noncontributory except for moderate hypertension treated with a loop diuretic and small dose of an ace inhibitor.

Physical examination showed a BP of 160/84, pulse 135, irregular. Cardiovascular examination revealed no murmurs or gallops.

An ECG was obtained, shown below.

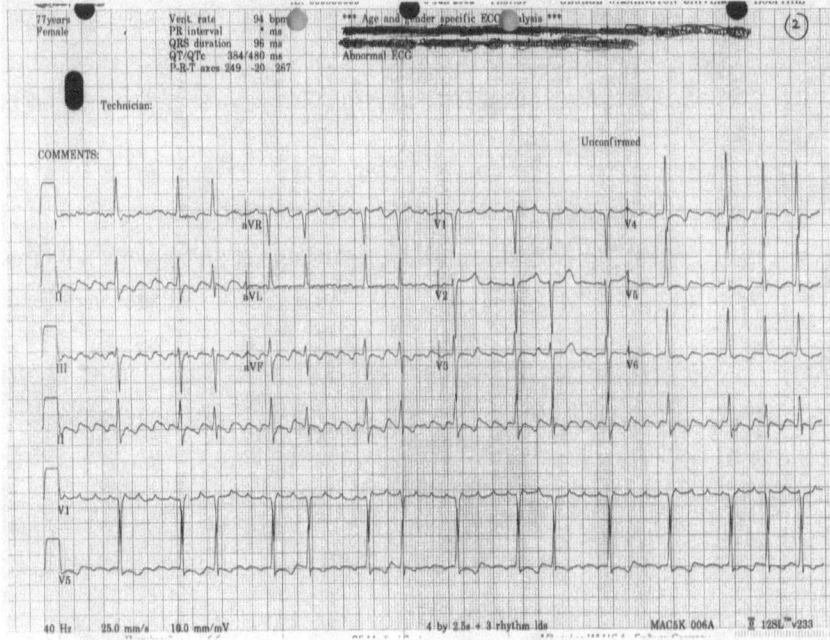

Fig. 32.1. ECG shows atrial fibrillation with variable ventricular response.

Initial treatment with a beta-blocker was instituted to control heart rate, and he was started on anticoagulants. After a few weeks and different attempts to control the arrhythmia, he was admitted for a therapeutic procedure.

The ECG show atrial fibrillation and an irregular ventricular rate of 90 beats per minute.

DISCUSSION

Some facts about trial fibrillation

- is the most common serious abnormal heart rhythm and.

- It affects 2% to 3% of the general population.

- The percentage of people with AF increases with age. The incidence is 0.14% for those under 50 years old, 4% for those between 60 and 70 years old, and 14% over 80 years old.

- Atrial fibrillation and resulted in 112,000 deaths in 2013, up from 29,000 in 1990. Increased longevity of the population ic considered the main factor in this increase.

The presentation of atrial fibrillation can differ from patient to patient. It may manifest with palpitations and the feeling of an irregular rhythm, while others will have worsening symptoms of heart failure, a stroke, or increased frequency of angina episodes.

What physiological changes occur as a result of atrial fibrillation?

- *Atrial activity becomes chaotic without a regular, functional atrial contraction.* This will do the following:
  - Increase blood stasis in the atria with the associated risk of clot formation. Most clots (90%) occur in the left atrial appendage.
  - *If untreated, the AV node may receive approximately 300 electrical impulses a minute, a rate that the node cannot transmit without resulting in a very rapid ventricular rate.* At this point, the AV node will demonstrate decremental conduction, with changes in the RR interval induced by the changing cycle length results in the irregularity of the rhythm.

- *In atrial fibrillation, the AV node refractory period will control the ventricular rate. If untreated, it will be fast.* If the patient is treated with a drug that decreases AV conduction velocity and increases refractory period (i.e., beta-blockers or calcium channel blockers), the ventricular rate will be slower.

- *In atrial fibrillation, the loss of P waves will translate in a reduction in ventricular filling and a decrease in cardiac output of approximately 20%.* This explains the onset of heart failure and the fatigue often reported by patients with atrial fibrillation.

- Additional consequences of atrial fibrillation are related to the abrupt decrease in cardiac output that

    - could decrease coronary blood flow, either initiating or worsening the symptoms of angina pectoris;

    - decrease cerebral blood flow resulting in transient ischemic attacks or causing strokes;

    - decrease renal flow and initiating renal failure; and

    - decrease mesenteric flow.

In addition to the consequences of decreased cardiac output, the increased risk of clot formation in the left atria can trigger embolic phenomena with the same physiological consequences.

Why does atrial fibrillation develop?

A prevalent theory is that the regular impulses produced by the sinus node for a normal heartbeat are overwhelmed by rapid electrical discharges produced in the atria and adjacent parts of the pulmonary veins. Sources of these disturbances are either automatic foci, often localized at one of the pulmonary veins, or a small number of localized sources in the form of either reentrant electrical spiral waves (rotors) or repetitive focal beats. These localized sources may be found in the left atrium near the pulmonary veins or in various other locations through both the left or right atrium.

Cardiopulmonary disease of any type increases the risk of atrial fibrillation.

- Valvular heart disease (such as mitral stenosis, mitral regurgitation, and tricuspid regurgitation).

- Hypertension.

- Congestive heart failure.

- Any inflammatory state that causes fibrosis of the atria.

- In elderly population, the increased number of amyloid deposits has been associated with atrial fibrillation.

- Mutation of the *lamin AC* gene is also associated with fibrosis of the atria that can lead to atrial fibrillation.

Regardless of etiology, progressive fibrosis and dilation of the atria are the common pathologic change. Once dilation of the atria has occurred, this begins a chain of events that leads to the activation of the renin-aldosterone-angiotensin system (RAAS) and subsequent increase in matrix metalloproteinases and disintegrin, which leads to atrial remodeling and fibrosis, with loss of atrial muscle mass.

TREATMENT

The treatment of atrial fibrillation can follow two different approaches:

- *Rhythm control.* Restoration of normal sinus rhythm is the goal, and this could be reached with the following:

    o **Drugs**
    - Sodium channel blockers which help the heart's rhythm by slowing the heart's ability to conduct electricity (flecainide, propafenone quinidine).
    - Potassium channel blockers slow down the number of electrical impulse (amiodarone, sotalol, dofetilide).

    o **Cardioversion**

    A single electrical shock that depolarizes the heart allows the dominant pacemaker, the sinus node, to regain control of the heart rhythm. Cardioversion is a time-honored procedure that is used less frequently since the availability of new drugs and the development of ablation.

    o **Ablation**

    Radiofrequency or criofrequency ablation are two methods used to create the scar point needed to control the fibrillatory impulses. After a single procedure, more than 50% of patients with an otherwise normal heart can enjoy freedom from arrhythmias. With two or more procedures, the efficacy can be as high as 80–90%. These results compare favorably with data on natural evolution of the disease or success observed with antiarrhythmic drugs and has become a favored approach in many cases.

- *Rate Control.* With this approach, the goal is to maintain ventricular rate between 60 and 80 beats per minute as well as a limited increase during moderate physical activity, increasing ventricular rate about 20% of the resting rate.

- *Anticoagulation.* The importance of anticoagulation must be emphasized. Because of the high risk of stroke, anticlotting medications are essential. Warfarin is preferred if valvular heart disease is the cause.

AF can be distinguished from atrial flutter (AFL), which appears as an organized electrical circuit usually in the right atrium.

CASE 32 QUESTIONS

See case 33.

CASE NO. 33: ATRIAL FLUTTER

A seventy-one-year-old retired physician presents to the office complaining of palpitations of about a twenty-four-hour duration. He describes them as the sudden onset of a rapid heart rate at 150 beats per minute and slight shortness of breath while climbing stairs.

His past medical history reveals a mitral and tricuspid valve repair for old rheumatic heart disease that had resulted in mitral regurgitation accompanied by significant tricuspid regurgitation.

Physical examination is as follows:

Left ventricular hypertrophy with apical impulse displaced to the left.

Auscultation demonstrates S1 is soft and a grade 2/6 pansystolic murmur at the apex radiating to the axilla. A grade 1/6 pansystolic murmur that increases with inspiration is best heard at the tricuspid area.

Pitting edema in feet and ankles is noted bilaterally.

The ECG is enclosed.

75 year old comes to the ED with shortness of breath and a rapid heart rate

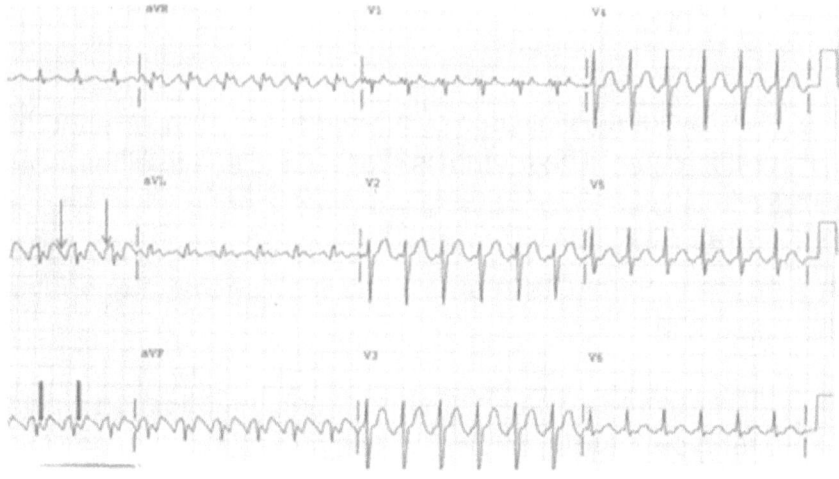

Fig. 33.1. Atrial rate is 300 per minute; ventricular rate is 150 per minute. Flutter waves are best seen in leads 2, 3 AVF.

DISCUSSION

Atrial flutter is often seen before the development of atrial fibrillation. Atrial flutter (see above) produces characteristic saw-toothed F waves of constant amplitude and an atrial rate of approximately 300 beats per minute.

An electrical impulse travels in a circular movement around the atrial myocardium. The ventricular rate is determined by the AV node refractory and is influenced by drugs that prolong it. Due to its longer refractory period, the AV node exerts a protective effect on heart rate by blocking atrial impulses exceeding about 180 beats/minute.

Although this abnormal heart rhythm typically occurs in individuals with cardiovascular disease (e.g., high blood pressure, coronary artery disease, and cardiomyopathy), it may occur spontaneously in people with otherwise normal hearts. It is typically not a stable rhythm and often degenerates into atrial fibrillation.

What is the mechanism?

Atrial flutter is initiated by a reentrant rhythm in either the right or left atrium. The rhythm is propagated due to differences in refractory periods of atrial tissue, that creates an electrical activity that moves in a self-perpetuating loop. Each cycle around the loop results in an electric impulse that propagates through the atria.

There are two types of atrial flutter, the common *type 1* and rarer *type 2*. Most individuals with atrial flutter will manifest only one of these.

Type 1. The reentrant loop circles the right atrium and passes through the lower atrium between the inferior vena cava and the tricuspid valve. The flutter waves in this rhythm are inverted in ECG leads 2, 3, and AVF.

Type 2. The flutter follows a significantly different reentry pathway to type 1 flutter and is typically faster, usually 340–440 beats per minute. It is common after incomplete left atrial ablation procedures.

TREATMENT

In general, atrial flutter should be managed the same as atrial fibrillation.

- *Rate control.* Since both atrial flutter and atrial fibrillation can be associated with very fast heart rates, both require medications such as beta-blockers or calcium channel blockers to decrease conduction through the AV node.

- *Rhythm control*
    - Restoration to normal sinus rhythm can be achieved in 70–90% with drugs such as ibutilide *or* dofetilide. Atrial flutter is less likely to convert than atrial fibrillation.
    - *Electrical conversion.* Atrial flutter is considerably more sensitive to electrical direct-current cardioversion than atrial fibrillation.
    - *Ablation.* Due to the reentrant nature of atrial flutter, it is often possible to ablate the circuit that causes atrial flutter with catheter ablation.
- *Anticoagulation.* Patients with atrial flutter, same as those with atrial fibrillation, require some form of anticoagulation or antiplatelet agent.

CASES 32–33 QUESTIONS

1. Ventricular rate in patients with atrial fibrillation is determined by

    a. Atrial rate
    b. Stroke volume
    c. Atrial volume
    d. AV node refractory period

2. Atrial fibrillation will affect

    a. End-diastolic volume
    b. Stroke volume
    c. Cardiac output
    d. All of the above

3. Atrial fibrillation originates from activity in the

    a. Right atrium
    b. Left atrial appendage
    c. Left atrial chamber
    d. Pulmonary veins

4. Cardioversion

    a. Prevents ventricular tachycardia
    b. Does not increase stroke risks
    c. Depolarizes only the atria
    d. May create brief period of asystole

5. Rate control eliminates the need for anticoagulation.

    a. True
    b. False

6. Anticoagulation before cardioversion is not necessary in atrial flutter.

    a. True
    b. False

7. Cardioversion of atrial flutter requires higher voltage that atrial fibrillation.

    a. True
    b. False

CASE NO. 34: LONG QT INTERVAL

TR, a twenty-five-year-old male, arrives to the ED indicating that he is feeling dizzy and his heart is beating very fast. A rhythm strip is obtained immediately.

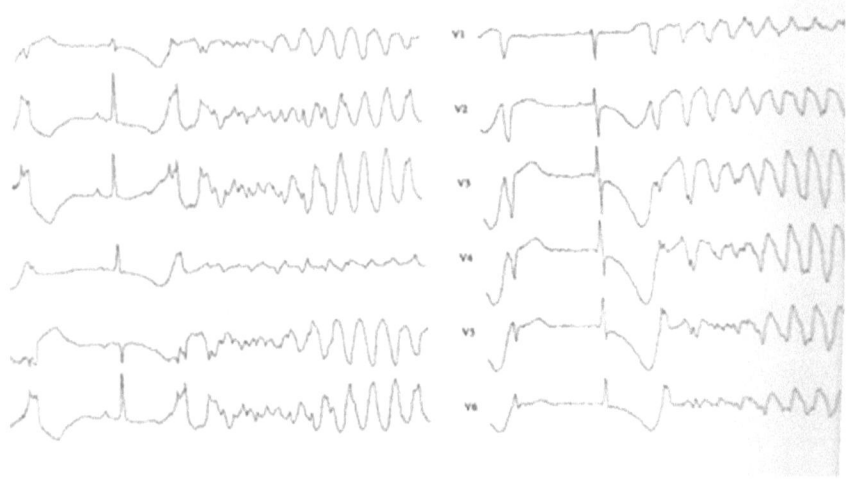

Fig. 34.1. The ECG reveals a ventricular rate of 300 beats per minute and the morphology with changing direction of the QRS commonly known as torsades de pointes.

Patient is treated and returns to normal sinus rhythm. He subsequently informed the physicians that he had been addicted to heroin and is now on treatment with methadone for the past few weeks.

His ECG is shown below.

24 y.o male. Longstanding Hx of heroin abuse. Mildly hyper

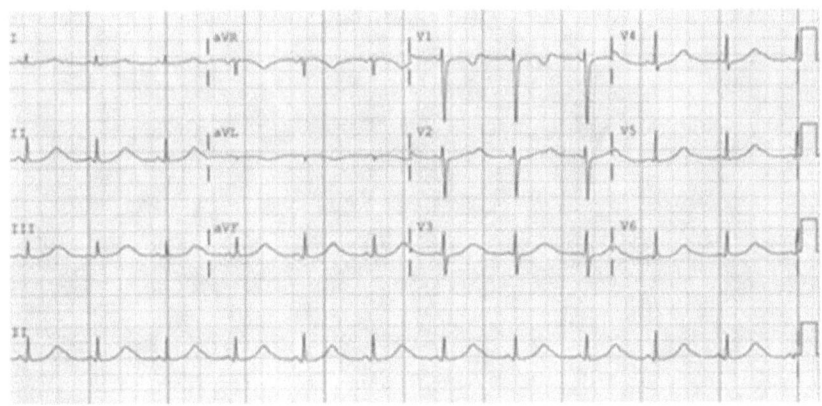

DISCUSSION

The arrhythmia presented by this patient is typical of ventricular tachycardia of the torsades de pointes type and associated with long QT intervals. A corrected Q-T interval (for heart rate) longer than 440 miliseconds is considered prolonged.

Long QT syndrome can arise from mutation of one of several genes that prolong the duration of the ventricular action potential

Inheritance of LQT syndrome can be in an autosomal dominant and less commonly in an autosomal recessive fashion. The autosomal recessive forms of LQTS tend to have a more severe phenotype, often associated with other congenital heart diseases, autism, immune deficiency and complex syndactyly (LQT8), or congenital neural deafness (LQT1).

A number of specific genes have been identified to be associated with LQTS.

LONG QT INTERVAL
Genomics, Risks and Treatment

NAME	GENE	ISSUE	THERAPY	% FAMILIAL	
LQT 1	KCNQ 1	Events during exercise	Avoid Competitive Sports	30-35%	K+ channel defect
LQT 2	KCNH 2	Auditory Stimulation Triggers	Beta Blocker therapy advised	25-30%	
LQT 3	SCN5A	Low risk with exercise Beta blockers cause high Mortality	Flecanide ICD	5-10%	Na+ channel defect
LQT 5	KCNE 1			< 1%	
LQT 6	KCNE 2			< 1%	

Ventricular tachycardia can develop spontaneously or be associated with a number of drugs as shown in the enclosed list.

DRUGS TO BE AVOIDED IN PATIENTS WITH LONG QT
(Partial List)

- Albuterol (bronchodilator)
- Amiodorone
- Amoxapine (antidepressant)
- Amphetamine
- Astemizole(antihistaminic)
- Clozapine (Anti-psychotic)
- Dopamine (Inotropic agent)
- Fluoxetine (Prozac)
- Mexiletine (antiarrhythmic)
- Salmeterol (COPD)
- Bepridil (antiangina)
- Chloroquine (antimalarial)
- Ciprofloxacin (antibiotic)
- Cisapride (GI)
- Clarithromycin (antibiotic)
- Ephedrine
- Epinephrine
- Erythromycin
- Methadone
- Lithium
- Oxytocin (Labor stimulation)

This arrhythmia is responsive to infusion of magnesium sulfate and may not be responsive to electrical cardioversion.

The most common causes of LQTS are mutations in the genes *KCNQ1* (LQT1), *KCNH2* (LQT2), and *SCN5A* (LQT3).

PATHOPHYSIOLOGY OF LONG QT SYNDROME

Long Q-T is associated with early afterdepolarizations that play a role in the development ventricular tachycardia After epolarization are oscillations in voltage oscillations that occur during the repolarizing phase of the cardiac action potential Early after depolarizations can trigger, ventricular tachycardia probably caused by reopening of calcium channels during the plateau of the action potential. An increased calcium filling of the sarcoplasmic reticulum may cause spontaneous calcium release during repolarization, resulting in a net depolarizing current.

Why can exercise cause the arrhythmia in predisposed subject? Adrenergic stimulation can increase the activity of these calcium channels,

TREATMENT

Patients with LQTS should be advised to avoid drugs that would prolong the QT interval. In addition, the following is important:

- **Arrhythmia prevention**

    These include administration of beta-receptor blocking agents, which decreases the risk of stress-induced arrhythmias. Beta-blockers are an effective treatment for LQTS caused by LQT1 and LQT2.

The use of should be considered when the QTc is greater than 500 msec and LQT2 and LQT3 genotypes are present.

- **Arrhythmia termination**

    Magnesium sulfate is often effective in terminating the arrhythmia.

    One effective form of arrhythmia termination in individuals with LQTS is placement of an implantable cardioverter-defibrillator (ICD. ICDs are commonly used in patients with fainting episodes despite beta-blocker therapy and in patients having experienced a cardiac arrest.

CASE 34 QUESTIONS

1. The following are risk factors for the development of torsades de pointes:

    a. Hypomagnesemia
    b. Hypokalemia
    c. Heart failure
    d. All of the above
    e. None of the above

2. In patients with torsades de pointes, in the following phase, the action potential is prolonged in

    a. Phase 0
    b. Phase 1
    c. Phase 2
    d. Phase 3
    e. Phase 4

3. The following drugs may be associated with long QT syndrome:

    a. Methadone
    b. Citalopram
    c. Cimetidine
    d. All of the above
    e. None of the above

4. One of the following may trigger an episode of ventricular tachycardia:

    a. Silence
    b. Sleep
    c. Noise
    d. Rest

5. Long QT syndrome can be

    a. Autosomal dominant
    b. Autosomal recessive
    c. Both
    d. Neither

CONGENITAL HEART DISEASE

CASE NO. 35: PATHOPHYSIOLOGY OF LEFT TO RIGHT SHUNTS—VENTRICULAR SEPTAL DEFECT

AT is a three-year-old girl brought in by her parents to evaluate a murmur detected at age one. The child is completely asymptomatic, active, and involved in normal child activities. Her growth and development are normal.

The murmur was first detected on a routine physical examination, and while they thought at the time it was a congenital heart lesion, the physician decided to wait because of the possibility that existed that the lesion (suspected to be a ventricular septal defect) could close on its own. Regular follow-up was advised.

Her growth and development was in the 92 percentile. The murmur was described as pansystolic, loudest over the tricuspid area and accompanied by a palpable thrill. There was no cyanosis, no evidence of ventricular hypertrophy or pulmonary hypertension, and all peripheral pulses were present and normal.

DISCUSSION

The case is illustrative of a ventricular septal defect without major hemodynamic consequences at the time of the physical examination. Distinctly, a left-to-right shunt was present.

Ventricular septal defect is the most common congenital cardiac anomaly in newborns and infants. Its prevalence is between 2 and 6 per 1,000 births, representing approximately 30–60% of all cardiac defects. The incidence in children and adults is much lower, suggesting that many defects, mainly the muscular or trabecular defects, close spontaneously after birth.

VSD occurs in three different locations:

- *Membranous.* They represent approximately 80% of all defects and are located in the membranous portion of the ventricular septum.
- *Ventricular septum.* Very common in newborns, they close spontaneously in the majority of cases. Represent 20% of all VSDs.
- *Supracristal.* This occur 5% above the crista supraventricularis of the right ventricle and often seen in tetralogy of Fallot.

What is the physiology of left-to-right shunts? What factors influence the magnitude of the shunt?

The magnitude of the left-to-right shunt is a function of the balance between systemic pressures/resistance and right-side pressure and resistance. The ratio is influenced by the physiological changes that occur after birth.

- *Major changes in circulation occur between fetal life and afterbirth that may delay the diagnosis until the newborn is several weeks old. In brief, the changes are as follows:*
    - During fetal life, oxygenated blood is delivered to the right atrium thu the umbilical vein. This blood then cross to the left side through an open septum secundum and the ductus arteriosus.

- Since the lungs are not inflated, pulmonary vascular resistance is high, limiting any potential of left-to-right shunts.

- At birth, lung expansion lowers pulmonary vascular resistance and pulmonary pressure. This normalization of pressures may take days or weeks, and it influences the relationship between left- and right-sided pressures and flow. Lowering of right-sided pressures will increase left-to-right shunt if a lesion exists.

- Left atrial pressure will increase as a result of the increased flow to the left atria, and the right atrial pressure may decrease as a result of the decreased right ventricular pressure. The above will lead to the closure of the foramen ovale by the septum secundum.

- The patient's ductus will close in the first month of life. The increased O_2 content will decrease, circulating prostaglandins and activating the muscular layer of the ductus, leading to its closure.

- By the fourth to sixth week, all these changes will be completed.

What determines the magnitude and direction of the left-to-right shunt in ventricular septal defect?

Blood will follow the path of least resistance. What influences the resistance to flow?

- ○ *The pressure difference (gradient) between left ventricle and right ventricle* This gradient is mainly systolic. During diastole, the pressure difference is minimal and is determined by ventricular compliance.

- ○ *The relationship between systemic and pulmonary vascular resistance*
  - If pulmonary resistance increases (i.e., pulmonary hypertension), the ratio between systemic and pulmonary resistances will decrease, and the shunt will decrease.
  - If systemic resistance decreases (for example, systemic hypotension), the ratio between systemic and pulmonary resistances will decrease, decreasing the shunt

- ○ *The size of the ventricular defect in relation to the size of the aortic outflow*
  - The size of an opening influences the resistance to flow. With a small defect in relation to the aortic outflow size, there will be greater resistance for flow through the defect and less resistance to flow through the aortic outflow, and the amount of shunt will decrease. The opposite will happen with large defects.

The physiological effects of left-to-right shunts are based on the amount of shunt flow. The consequences are as follows:

- *Left ventricular hypertrophy that may lead to heart failure.* The left ventricle will be tasked with increased work, having to maintain an adequate cardiac output and dealing with the increased volume that will move to the right ventricle through the defect. This will result in an increase in left ventricular end-diastolic volume.

- *Ventricular contractility will increase.* This results in a slight rise in systolic pressure, a faster rise in ventricular and arterial pressure, and an *increase in ventricular work*. These changes may have clinical consequences, especially in children with large defects.

- *Pulmonary hypertension.* This is the most serious consequence of the left-to-right shunt. The mechanism is not clear, but a very likely mechanism is the increase in flow that may damage the pulmonary vessel endothelium and release substances such as endothelin that causes vasoconstriction. The pulmonary vasoconstriction can, over time, lead to hypertrophy of the muscular layer and other pathological changes, causing severe pulmonary hypertension.

- *Right ventricular hypertension and hypertrophy.* Pulmonary hypertension can result in a major increase in right ventricular pressure and ventricular hypertrophy that eventually may reverse the shunt to a right-to-left shunt.

- *Right ventricular pressure may reach systemic levels.* The shunt may become bidirectional as a result in timing differences and changes in compliance.

The physical findings influenced by the amount of shunt are as follows:

- *Systolic murmur.* The murmur's intensity and duration are determined by the pressure gradient between the left and right ventricle. When pulmonary hypertension develops, the intensity of the murmur will decrease.

- *S3 and mitral diastolic rumble.* The volume of shunted blood that will return to the left atria will increase, flow through the mitral valve, and create vibrations that result in a soft apical diastolic murmur. This is observed when the shunt results in pulmonary flow being twice of systemic flow.

- *Loud P2.* Prominent as pulmonary hypertension develops.

TREATMENT

Treatment of a VSD requires closure of the defect. Closure of the defect can be achieved by the following:

- *Device implantation.* At present, this is limited to muscular type VSD, where closure can be obtained via a cardiac catheterization and insertion of a closure device.
- *Cardiac surgery.* Surgical closure of a membranous VSD is performed on cardiopulmonary bypass with ischemic arrest using patch materials such as native pericardium, bovine pericardium, Gore-Tex, or Dacron. Critical attention is necessary to avoid injury to the conduction system located and the aortic valve.

CASE 35 QUESTIONS

1. Systemic hypotension

    a. Decreases left/right pressure gradient
    b. Increases left-to-right shunts
    c. May not cause cyanosis
    d. Increase arterial O_2 saturation

2. Pulmonary hypertension in congenital heart disease

    a. May decrease arterial O_2 saturation
    b. Is caused by increased pulmonary resistance
    c. Results from pulmonary arterial intimal damage
    d. All of the above
    e. None of the above

3. In reference to membranous defects, it

    a. Is the most common type of VSD
    b. Cannot spontaneously close
    c. Will always cause endocarditis
    d. Rarely causes pulmonary hypertension

4. The magnitude of the left-to-right shunt

    a. Will be influenced by the type of defect
    b. Will be influenced by size of the defect
    c. Will be influenced by pulmonary pressure
    d. All of the above
    e. None of the above

5. Supracristal defects

    a. Are the most common types of VSD
    b. Are most often associated with other defects
    c. Will never cause pulmonary hypertension
    d. Will commonly cause endocarditis

CASE NO. 36: ATRIAL SEPTAL DEFECT

Ms. SM, a twenty-eight-year-old female, was referred for evaluation of a cardiac murmur. At age twelve, her parents were told she had a heart murmur, considered to be a physiologic murmur.

She was free of symptoms and lived a very active life. An avid runner and tennis player, she never complained of exercise-related shortness of breath, palpitations, or chest pain.

Her cardiovascular examination revealed normal JVP. All arterial pulses were present and normal.

There was no evidence of cardiomegaly. No thrills were detected.

First heart sound was normal, and second heart sound had fixed splitting.

A grade 3 ejection systolic murmur was audible over the pulmonic area, and a soft diastolic rumble was heard over the tricuspid area that followed an S3.

DISCUSSION

Atrial septal defect (ASD) is one of the most common congenital cardiac defects. There are several different types of atrial septal defect:

- *Ostium secundum ASD*. It results from excessive reabsorption of the septum primum or a large foramen ovale. They account for 70–75% of all cases of ASD, representing approximately 6–10% of all congenital cardiac defects and 30–40% of all congenital heart diseases in patients older than forty years.

- *Ostium primum ASD.* This is caused by incomplete fusion of septum primum with the endocardial cushions, and it lies immediately adjacent to the atrioventricular (AV) valves. In most cases, only the anterior leaflet of the mitral valve is displaced, and it is commonly cleft, resulting also in mitral regurgitation.

- *Sinus venosus ASD.* This type of defect is the least common of the three, seen in 5–10% of all ASDs. The defect is located in the superior aspect of the atrial septum and is often associated with an anomalous connection of the pulmonary veins.

- *Coronary sinus ASD.* Coronary sinus defect is characterized by unroofed coronary sinus and persistent left superior vena cava that drains into the left atrium and can result in desaturation due to right-to-left shunt into the left atrium.

ASD occurs with a female-to-male ratio of approximately 2:1.

Patients with ASD can be asymptomatic through infancy and childhood, depending on the magnitude of the left-to-right shunt. Symptoms become more common with advancing age, and by age forty, 90% of untreated patients have symptoms of exertional dyspnea, fatigue, palpitation, sustained arrhythmias, or even evidence of heart failure

What is the physiology of the left-to right-shunt in ASD?

The shunt occurs primarily during late systole and early diastole and is influenced by the difference in compliance between the right and left ventricles. The right ventricle compliance is lower than the left ventricle and is an important factor in determining the amount of shunt.

As consequences of the left-to-right shunt, RV volume is increased and right ventricular work is increased

The shunt increases right chamber volume and flow and influences the auscultatory findings, as follows:

- *Fixed splitting of the second heart sound.* A characteristic physical finding is caused by the following:
    - Increased duration of right ventricular systole because of the increased volume of the RV.
    - The RV volume remains elevated both in inspiration and expiration. RV compliance determines the volume capacity of the RV.
    - The source of the shunted blood changes. During inspiration, there will be more venous return, and during expiration, there will be more flow from the left atria. The duration of systole is fixed by the increased volume and limited compliance of the right ventricle, explaining the lack of respiratory changes in RV systole.
- *The ejection systolic murmur* is caused by the turbulence created by the increase stroke volume from the right ventricle.
- *The diastolic rumble following an S3* results from the increased flow across the tricuspid valve.

The defects may remain asymptomatic until the fourth decade when symptoms associated with the development of pulmonary hypertension appear.

TREATMENT

Closure of the ASD is the only treatment. Many defects may require surgery, or many can be corrected with a devise inserted via a catheter.

Surgical mortality due to closure of an ASD is lowest when the procedure is performed prior to the development of significant pulmonary hypertension. The lowest mortality rates are achieved in individuals with a pulmonary artery systolic pressure less than 40 mm Hg.

CASE 36 QUESTIONS

1. In a patient with a ostium primum defect, very often there is

    a. Deformity in the mitral valve
    b. Deformity in the tricuspid valve
    c. Myocardial involvement
    d. Increased clot formation in the right ventricle

2. In patients with ASD

    a. Right ventricular compliance is increased
    b. Pulmonary venous return is decreased
    c. Left atrial volume is decreased
    d. Right ventricular stroke volume is decreased

3. The most common type of ASD is

    a. Sinus venous
    b. Primum defect
    c. Secundum defect
    d. Coronary sinus defect

4. Foramen ovale

    a. Is always patent
    b. Can cause paradoxical embolus
    c. Is always associated with coronary sinus defects
    d. Is always associated with sinus venosus defects

5. Abnormal insertion of the superior vena cava is seen in

    a. Primum defects
    b. Secundum defects
    c. Coronary sinus defects
    d. Sinus venosus defects

CASE NO. 37: PATENT DUCTUS ARTERIOSUS

A second year medical student is asked to examine a four-month-old infant brought by the mother to the cardiology clinic for evaluation of a cardiac murmur recently noted. Mother indicates that the child's growth and development are normal, growing and gaining weight.

On physical examination, he appears to be developing normally. All peripheral pulses are normal. There is no cyanosis. There is no evidence of either left or right biventricular hypertrophy.

On auscultation, heart sounds are normal. A grade 3/6 continuous murmur is best heard over the pulmonic area and radiating through the precordium.

A chest x-ray is compatible with a left-to-right shunt, and the ECG is normal.

The diagnosis of patent ductus arteriosus is made.

DISCUSSION

Some facts about the ductus arteriosus

- Is a communication between the pulmonary and systemic circulation, essential during intrauterine
- Originates from the sixth aortic arch
- After birth, pO_2 rises, resulting in a marked drop in circulating prostaglandins that cause
- The increased pO2 increases contraction of the muscle layers and the ductus leading to its spontaneous closure.
- Closure happens usually during the first month of life.

- The estimated incidence of patent ductus arteriosus (PDA) in US children born at term is between 0.02% and 0.006% of live births.
- The incidence is increased in children who are born prematurely, 20% in premature infants born at 32 weeks' gestation, and up to 60% in those with gestation less than twenty-eight weeks.
- Children with a history of perinatal asphyxia, born at high altitude and up to 30% of low birth weight infants (< 2,500 g), often retain an open patent ductus arteriosus.

What are some of the physiological changes at birth?

At birth, the following takes place:

- The placenta is removed, eliminating a major source of prostaglandin production.
- The lungs expand, activating the organ in which most prostaglandins are metabolized.
- With the onset of normal respiration, oxygen tension in the blood markedly increases.
- Lung expansion causes a decrease in pulmonary vascular resistance, increasing the pressure differential between left and right circulations that will determine presence and magnitude of the shunt.

What is the pathophysiology associated with a PDA?

If the ductus remains patent, it creates a *left-to-right shunt*. The volume of the shunt is determined by

- the pressure gradient between systemic and pulmonary circuits, which, in turn, are influenced by
- the diameter and length of the ductus and

- the pulmonary vascular resistance (PVR).

The shunt causes an increase in end-diastolic volume that may lead to left ventricular hypertrophy and, if the shunt is very large, to left ventricular failure.

The magnitude of the left-to-right shunt can induce pulmonary vasoconstriction, leading to pulmonary hypertension as discussed in a previous section.

Persistence of an open ductus with its associated physiological changes will result in the following physical findings:

- A continuous murmur resulting from turbulence through the ductus during both systole and diastole.
- A displaced apical impulse if left ventricular hypertrophy occurs.
- Increased ventricular contractility as volume increases.
- Ventricular work increases.
- Larger flow returning to the left atria. The large flow causes turbulence and, often, a diastolic murmur across the mitral valve.

The most serious complication is the evolution from reactive pulmonary hypertension to fixed or permanent pulmonary hypertension, as it can occur in all lesions with large left-to-right shunts. The result will be right ventricular hypertension and hypertrophy that will have a loud P2 as well as the clinical manifestations discussed earlier.

TREATMENT

The therapeutic goal is to eliminate the shunt, thus preventing

- left heart hypertrophy and failure,
- pulmonary hypertension, and
- infective endocarditis.

Prostaglandins are responsible for keeping the ductus open, thus NSAIDS, such as indomethacin, which can inhibit prostaglandin synthesis, have been used to initiate PDA closure.

More recently, PDAs can be closed by percutaneous interventional method (avoiding open-heart surgery). A platinum coil or an occluder device can be deployed via a catheter through the femoral vein or femoral artery. If a child is born with a ventricular septal defect as he grows, a left-to-right shunt will be present.

CASE 37 QUESTIONS

1. If a patient with a PDA develops significant pulmonary hypertension

    a. Diastolic shunt decreases
    b. O_2 saturation in lower extremities decreases
    c. Diastolic component of the murmur may disappear
    d. All of the above
    e. None of the above

2. The PDA originates from

    a. Right fourth aortic arch
    b. Left sixth aortic arch
    c. Fourth aortic arch
    d. Third aortic arch

3. A PDA with a large left-to-right shunt can cause

    a. Diastolic rumble through the mitral valve
    b. Diastolic rumble through the tricuspid valve
    c. Aortic diastolic murmur
    d. Mitral pansystolic murmur

4. Closure of the ductus occurs in the

    a. First year of life
    b. First week of life
    c. First month of life
    d. First day of life

5. Closure of the ductus is associated with

    a. Increased prostaglandins after birth
    b. Growth in PDA endothelium
    c. Decreased prostaglandins after birth
    d. Decreased arterial O_2

CASE NO. 38: CONGENITAL CARDIAC DEFECT AND PULMONARY HYPERTENSION

A third year medical student is assigned to a congenital heart disease clinic and is asked to interview and examine a forty-two-year-old lady who reports the following:

- At age seventeen, she was diagnosed as being born with an atrial septal defect, but her family, for cultural and religious reasons, refused to consent for further diagnostic procedures or an eventual heart surgery to repair the defect.
- She had been asymptomatic until seven years ago when she noticed progressive shortness of breath on moderate activity. Also she noted that her lips and fingernails turned blue, first after exercise and currently all the time. She also reports one fainting episode that occurred after having to climb several flights of stairs.

Physical examination reveals

- a well-developed and nourished female with no respiratory distress at rest and
- cyanosis of lips and fingernails and slight clubbing of fingers.

Cardiovascular examination shows

- a distended jugular vein with a prominent "a" wave,
- a palpable and sustained parasternal lift,
- a loud pulmonary component of P2, and
- a grade 2/6 systolic murmur at the left intercostal space.

The ECG showed right axis deviation and evidence of right ventricular hypertrophy.

Chest x-ray demonstrates dry lung fields and a large pulmonary artery.

DISCUSSION

This case exemplifies an untreated congenital heart lesion that develops progressive pulmonary hypertension concluding in a classical example of Eisenmenger syndrome.

When does pulmonary hypertension develop in subjects with congenital heart disease?

As shown in the enclosed table, age of development of pulmonary hypertension is influenced by the type of defect, the amount of shunt, and the size of the defect. Large ventricular septal defects may lead to pulmonary hypertension early in life. Characteristically, patients with atrial septal defect will not have serious pulmonary hypertension until the fourth decade.

DEVELOPMENT OF EISENMENGER BY AGE AND DEFECT *(% by diagnosis)*

	PDA	VSD	ASD
INFANCY	79	83	8
CHILDHOOD	4	15	
ADULTS	17	2	92

The shunt volume as well as the pressure associated with the type of lesion partially explain the differences in the development of Eisenmenger syndrome.

What is the prognosis of Eisenmenger syndrome?

SURVIVAL TO AGE

20........................100%

40.........................94%

60.........................52%

What is the pathophysiology of pulmonary hypertension in congenital heart disease with left-to-right shunts?

The mediators that regulate the diameter of the pulmonary vessel include nitrous oxide and prostacyclin that induce vasodilatation and endothelin -1, which induces vasoconstriction. All three mediators may be present to maintain pulmonary vascular tone at an optimal level. Increases or decreases in the amounts of any one agent they stimulate and alter the balance toward vasodilation or vasoconstriction.

The initial step in the development of pulmonary hypertension is related to the high flow that that will cause endothelial damage and the release of endothelin and the resulting vasoconstriction.

The changes in pressure that resulted from the vasoconstriction are explained by the Poiseuille law (resistance to flow in a tube is equal to the product of the length of the tube and the fourth power of the internal radius of the tube). A small change in the radius of the vessel will have a significant change in the resistance to flow and the ensuing increase in pressure.

Some consequences follow the vasoconstriction. The initial vasoconstriction (reactive pulmonary hypertension) will eventually lead to fixed pulmonary hypertension with medial hypertrophy, concentric nonlaminar intimal fibrosis, eccentric intimal fibrosis, and thrombotic lesions.

What is the mechanism of cyanosis in patients with Eisenmenger syndrome?

- *Central cyanosis.* It develops when arterial oxygen saturation drops to ≤ 85% or ≤ 75%. Pulmonary hypertension results in shunt reversal and the resulting increased mixture of oxygenated and unoxygenated blood.

- *Peripheral cyanosis.* This results in lower cardiac output commonly caused by the pulmonary hypertension and the associated decreased preload.

  In patients with shunts and pulmonary hypertension, the mechanism of cyanosis is combined.

TREATMENT

Since the development of several new drugs, the treatment of pulmonary hypertension has improved dramatically in the last decade. The goals of modern medical treatment are to obtain vasodilatation of the pulmonary arteries to lower pressure, to maintain oxygen content, and to prevent clot formation in pulmonary arteries.

- **Blood vessel dilators (vasodilators)**
    - *Epoprostenol.* One of the most commonly prescribed vasodilators. The drawback is that its effects last only a few minutes, and the drug must

be continuously injected through an intravenous (IV) catheter.

- *Iloprotst.* Another form of the drug that can be inhaled six to nine times a day through a nebulizer.

- *Treprostinil.* Can be given four times a day. It can be inhaled, taken as oral medication, or administered by injection.

- **Endothelin receptor antagonists**

  These medications reverse the effect of endothelin. They include bosentan, macitentan, and ambrisentan.

  - *Sildenafil and tadalafil.* These are sometimes used to treat pulmonary hypertension. These drugs work through their vasodilating effect.

  - *High-dose calcium channel blockers.* Also acting as vasodilators, they include medications such as amlodipine, diltiazem, and nifedipine. Although calcium channel blockers can be effective, only a small number of people with pulmonary hypertension respond to them.

  - *Soluble guanylate cyclase (SGC) stimulator.* Soluble guanylate cyclase (SGC) stimulators interact with nitric oxide and help relax the pulmonary arteries and lower the pressure within the arteries.

- **Anticoagulants**

  These prevent the formation of blood clots within the small pulmonary arteries.

- **Oxygen**

- **Surgeries**

    - *Atrial septostomy.* An opening between the upper left and right atria can relieve the pressure on the right side of your heart but causes right-to-left shunt.

    - *Transplantation.* In some cases, a lung or heart-lung transplant might be an option, especially for younger people.

CASE 38 QUESTIONS

1. In patients with congenital heart disease, the development of pulmonary hypertension is usually related to

    a. Cyanosis
    b. Decreased systemic resistance
    c. Pulmonary vasoconstriction
    d. Hypoventilation

2. In patients with congenital heart diseases

    a. Pulmonary hypertension is always reversible
    b. Pulmonary resistance will be normal
    c. Right-to-left shunt will only be diastolic
    d. Will not be responsive to drugs

3. The following drugs may lower pulmonary pressure:

    a. Isoproterenol
    b. Hydrochlorothiazide
    c. Bosentan
    d. Aspirin

4. One of the following drugs may lower pulmonary pressure:

    a. Digoxin
    b. Ibuprofen
    c. Sildenafil
    d. Warfarin

5. In a patient with VSD and pulmonary hypertension, a severe drop in systemic pressure can

    a. Lower O_2 saturation
    b. Increase left-to-right shunt
    c. Lower arterial pH
    d. Decrease pulmonary resistance

CASE NO. 39: CYANOTIC HEART DISEASE— TETRALOGY OF FALLOT

A twenty-seven-year-old lady delivers a six-pound baby boy after an uncomplicated labor and delivery. The baby appears normal, although both nurses and pediatrician noted he was cyanotic. In a few hours, he is evaluated by a pediatric cardiologist who determines that the child was born with a cyanotic heart disease, most likely tetralogy of Fallot.

Further diagnostic studies confirm the original clinical suspicion

DISCUSSION

Tetralogy of Fallot (TOF) is the most common cause of cyanotic congenital heart disease accounting for one-third of all CHD in patients younger than fifteen years.

Some facts about Tetralogy of Fallot

- represents approximately 10% of cases of congenital heart disease (CHD), and it occurs in 3–6 infants for every 10,000 births
- higher incidence is seen in children of women who had maternal rubella (or other viral illnesses) during pregnancy or had poor prenatal nutrition, maternal alcohol use, maternal age older than forty years, maternal phenylketonuria and diabetes.
- Children with Down syndrome also have a higher incidence of tetralogy of Fallot, as do infants with fetal hydantoin syndrome or fetal carbamazepine syndrome.
- Embryologically, is a malformation of the conotruncal region

- can be associated with a number of other lesions such abnormal facies, cleft palate, or hypocalcemia, as well as other cardiac defects.

Classically, in tetralogy, there are four defects:

- *Ventricular septal defect.* The defect is usually posterior and superior to the crista supraventricularis of the right ventricle. In the majority of cases, it is single and large.

- *Pulmonary stenosis.* It can occur at the pulmonary valve (valvular stenosis) or just below the pulmonary valve (infundibular stenosis). Atresia of the pulmonary artery is also seen. The pulmonic stenosis is the most significant of the anomalies, with the other associated malformations acting as compensatory mechanisms. The degree of stenosis varies between individuals and is the primary determinant of symptoms and severity.

- *Right ventricular hypertrophy.* A consequence of the pulmonic stenosis. This feature is now generally agreed to be a secondary anomaly.

- *Overriding aorta.* This causes the right-to-left shunt. A biventricular connection of the aorta that is situated above the ventricular septal defect. The degree to which the aorta is attached to the right ventricle is referred to as its degree of override. The aortic root can be displaced toward the front (anteriorly) or directly above the septal defect, but it is always abnormally located to the right of the root of the pulmonary artery. The degree of override is extremely variable, with 5–95% of the valve being connected to the right ventricle.

Additional lesions may include

- a patent foramen ovale or atrial septal defect (pentalogy of Fallot);
- a bicuspid pulmonary valve, in 60%;
- an atrioventricular septal defect;
- coronary artery anomalies, in 10%;
- partially or totally anomalous pulmonary venous return;
- right-sided aortic arch, in 25%; and
- stenosis of the left pulmonary artery, in 40%.

THE PATHOPHYSIOLOGY OF TETRALOGY OF FALLOT

The pulmonic stenosis creates the elevation or right ventricular pressure that causes the right-to-left shunt through the VSD. The magnitude of the shunt is determined by which of the lesions predominate and are responsible for the degree and severity of the condition.

The right and left circuits face different levels of resistance, and the balance between the two will be what determines the shunting.

- If the pulmonic stenosis is severe and the VSD large, then the right-to-left shunt is facilitated.
- If the pulmonic stenosis is mild, resistance to flow will not be as major and magnitude of cyanosis is less.

In addition, the degree of overriding of the aorta will influence the magnitude of the right-to-left shunt.

What are the complications of right-to-left shunts?

- *Clubbing.* Clubbing is a common finding in patients with right-to-left shunts and is also seen in patients with COPD, lung cancer, and liver cirrhosis.

  Clubbing results from alterations in size and configuration of the clubbed nail bed, beginning with increased interstitial edema. As clubbing progresses, the volume of the terminal portion of the digit may increase because of an increase in the vascular connective tissue.

- *Paradoxical embolization.* This is caused by a blood clot, commonly originating from the lower extremities, that traverses from right to left through the existing communication.

  Such an event may cause

  - strokes and
  - brain abscesses.

- *Hypoxic spells.* These are caused by any decrease in peripheral vascular resistance that facilitates the increase of right-to-left shunting. This is common in patients with tetralogy of Fallot but may also happen in patients with Eisenmenger, secondary to other congenital lesions.

  There are two mechanisms for the hypoxic spells:

  - In patients with tetralogy, the common mechanism is a further increase in right ventricular outflow obstruction secondary to increased contractility.
  - Another mechanism is associated with exercise that lowers systemic resistance, and the

increased imbalance between pulmonary and systemic resistance increases right-to-left shunt and markedly lowers O_2 saturation.

Squatting. This is also common in subjects with tetralogy of Fallot. Squatting results in increased peripheral vascular resistance, elevating systemic pressure and altering the relationship between systemic and pulmonary resistances, causing a decrease in right-to-left shunt and improvement in O_2 saturation

TREATMENT

Surgical repair is the only alternative. At present, correction of tetralogy can be performed in children under one year with a perioperative mortality of 5%.

CASE 39 QUESTIONS

1. In tetralogy, the VSD

    a. Will spontaneously close
    b. Involve the membranous septum
    c. Is commonly located above the crista supraventricularis
    d. Atrial septal defect is always present

2. The severity of the pulmonic stenosis

    a. Will influence O2 saturation
    b. Will only involve the valve
    c. Only affects the pulmonary arteries
    d. Cannot involve the outflow of the RV

3. The overriding of the aorta

    a. May affect O_2 saturation
    b. Is always located to the left of the pulmonary arteries
    c. Is not important in the clinical presentation
    d. The aortic root is always displaced posteriorly

4. In TOF, the following defects are common:

    a. Aortic stenosis
    b. Transposition of the great vessels
    c. Stenosis of the left pulmonary artery
    d. Anomalous pulmonary venous drainage

5. Squatting will

    a. Increase right-to-left shunt
    b. Decrease pulmonary resistance
    c. Increase systemic resistance
    d. Decrease O_2 saturation

CASE NO. 40: PULMONARY STENOSIS

A ten-year-old girl is referred by her pediatrician for evaluation of a heart murmur that he detected on a routine annual physical for school. She was a new patient since the family only recently moved to town. The mother had no knowledge of this murmur.

The patient had a normal childhood with normal growth and development and had all the pertinent vaccination.

Physical examination revealed a well-nourished and developed girl in no distress. Height and weight were within the 95th percentile for her age.

There was no cyanosis or clubbing. All peripheral pulses were normal.

Cardiovascular examination demonstrated the following:

- Normal JVP
- Strong parasternal lift, suggestive of right ventricular hypertrophy
- No thrills
- Auscultation:
    - Normal S1 and S2 with normal splitting
    - Ejection sound on second left space
    - S3
    - Grade 3/6 ejection systolic murmur best heard on pulmonic area

Remaining of the physical examination was normal.

ECG and chest x-ray were normal.

DISCUSSION

The presence of this systolic murmur with no other significant findings brings out a differential between functional murmur and some mild right ventricular outflow obstruction such as pulmonic stenosis.

- **Pulmonic stenosis** is usually due to isolated valvular obstruction (pulmonary valve stenosis), but it may be due to subvalvular or supravalvular obstruction, such as infundibular stenosis. It may occur in association with other congenital heart defects as part of more complicated syndromes (for example, tetralogy of Fallot).

    A stenotic pulmonary valve usually occurs without associated congenital abnormalities, although it may be associated with other structural abnormalities of the heart (i.e., tetralogy of Fallot).

Isolated valvular PS comprises approximately 10% of all congenital heart diseases. Typically, the valve commissures are partially fused, and the three leaflets are thin and pliant, resulting in a conical or dome-shaped structure with a narrowed central orifice. Poststenotic pulmonary artery dilatation may occur owing to "jet-effect" hemodynamics.

Alternatively, approximately 10–15% of individuals with valvular PS have leaflets irregularly shaped and thickened, with little fusion and reduced mobility. The leaflets are composed of myxomatous tissue, the valve annulus is usually small, and the supravalvular area of the pulmonary trunk is usually hypoplastic.

A bicuspid valve is found in as many as 90% of patients with tetralogy of Fallot.

The pulmonary valve area of a healthy adult is 2.0 cm²/m² of the body surface area.

- Mild valvular PS is defined by a valve area larger than 1 cm² and a transvalvular pressure gradient of less than 50 mm Hg.
- Moderately severe PS occurs if the valve area is 0.5–1.0 cm², with a transvalvular pressure gradient between 50 and 75 mm Hg.
- Severe PS is defined by a valve area smaller than 0.5 cm² and a transvalvular pressure gradient greater than 75 mm Hg.

The following are some characteristic findings of valvular PS:

   ○ Parasternal lift as a function of the severity of the right ventricular hypertrophy
   ○ Palpable thrill, second left interspace, determined by the severity of the gradient
   ○ Ejection click if leaflets are mobile
   ○ Ejection systolic murmur at second left interspace

- **Congenital stenosis of the pulmonary artery branches** is an anomaly characterized by narrowed segments of one or more of the main or peripheral branches of the pulmonary artery. It is relatively uncommon, and it represents 3% of all congenital heart diseases.

The obstruction may be locked in the periphery of the branches, in either the left or right pulmonary arteries or in the main trunk. The multiple possibilities reflect the embryology of the arteries. The main trunk originates from the truncus arteriosus, the right and left branches originate from the sixth aortic arch, and the peripheral arteries originate from the development of the lungs.

Pulmonary valve stenosis has a very good prognosis and is often treated with angioplasty.

Pulmonary branch stenosis also has a good prognosis and rarely requires surgical repair—this being difficult if there are several stenotic areas in peripheral branches.

CASE 40 QUESTIONS

1. Pulmonary branch stenosis is related to the following maternal infection during pregnancy:

    a. Polio
    b. Influenza
    c. Rubella
    d. All or the above

2. Bicuspid pulmonic stenosis is rare in tetralogy of Fallot

    a. True
    b. False

3. Pulmonary stenosis

    a. Increases LV preload
    b. Decreases LV preload
    c. Increases LV volume
    d. All of the above

CORRECT ANSWERS

The following are the correct answers:

CASE 1 = 1-b, 2-b, 3-b, 4-d, 5-b, 6-c, 7-c

CASE 2 = 1-d, 2-b, 3-c, 4-b, 5-a, 6-a

CASE 3 = 1-d, 2-b, 3-c, 4- a, 5-b, 6-b, 7-a

CASE 4 = 1-b, 2-a, 3-b, 4-b, 5-a, 6-c, 7-c

CASE 5 = 1-c, 2-b, 3-a, 4-a

CASE 6 = 1-c, 2-b, 3-c, 4-b

CASE 7 = 1-a, 2-a, 3-c, 4-b, 5-b, 6-b

CASE 8 = 1-c, 2-b, 3-c, 4-c

CASE 9 = 1-b, 2-d, 3-d, 4-c, 5-c

CASE 10 = 1-b, 2-c, 3-a, 4-c, 5-d, 6-b

CASE 11 = 1-d, 2-d, 3-c, 4-d, 5-c

CASE 12 = 1-d, 2-c, 3-c, 4-c, 5-, 6-d

CASE 13 = 1-b, 2-e, 3a, 4-c, 5-c

CASE 14 = 1-c, 2-b, 3-b, 4-b

CASE 15 = 1-b, 2-b, 3-c, 4-c, 5-b, 6-c

CASE 16 = 1-c, 2-a, 3-b, 4-b, 5-c

CASE 17 = 1-d, 2-c, 3-c, 4-?, 5-d

CASE 18 = 1-a, 2-c, 3-b, 4-b, 5-a

CASE 19 = 1-d, 2-c, 3-d, 4-d, 5-d

CASE 20 = 1-c, 2-b, 3-a, 4-c, 5-?, 6-c

CASE 21 = 1-c, 2-d, 3-a, 4-c, 5-d,

CASE 22 = 1-c, 2-b, 3-d, 4-a, 5-b

CASE 23 = 1-c, 2-b, 3-c, 4-c

CASE 24 = 1-a, 2-c, 3-c, 4-c, 5-a, 6-d

CASE 25 = 1-c, 2-b, 3-d, 4-c, 5-d, 6-c,

CASE 26 = 1-a, 2-c, 3-a, 4-e, 5-b

CASE 27 = 1-b, 2-c, 3-d, 4-b

CASE28 = 1-c, 2-b, 3-b, 4-b,

CASE 29 = 1-c, 2-b, 3-d, 4-c, 5-d, 6-c

CASE 30 = 1-d, 2-a, 3-a, 4-b, 5-c,

CASE 31 = 1-b, 2-b, 3-d, 4-b

CASE 32–33 = 1-d, 2-d, 3-d, 4-d, 5-b, 6-b, 7-b

CASE 34 = 1-a, 2-d, 3-d, 4-c, 5-c

CASE 35 = 1-a, 2-d, 3-a, 4-d, 5-b

CASE 36 = 1-a, 2-d, 3-c, 4-b, 5-c

CASE 37 = 1-d, 2-b, 3-a, 4-c, 5-c

CASE 38 = 1-c, 2-b, 3-c, 4-c, 5-a

CASE 39 = 1-c, 2-a, 3-a, 4-c, 5-c

CASE 40 = 1-c, 2-b, 3-b

SELECTED REFERENCES

BOOKS

Alpert JS, Sabik J, Cosgrove DM III. Mitral valve disease. In: Textbook of Cardiovascular Medicine, Topol EJ (Ed), Lippincott-Raven, Philadelphia 1998. p.503

Braunwald E. *Heart Disease: A Textbook of Cardiovascular Medicine*. 10th ed. Philadelphia, Pa: Elsevier Saunders; 2015.

Crowley, Leonard V. An Introduction to Human Disease: Pathology and Pathophysiology Correlations. *Jones & Bartlett Publishers. p. 323.*

Guyton, A John E. *Textbook of medical physiology* (11th ed.). Philadelphia: W.B. Saunders

Harrison's principles of internal medicine. *New York: McGraw-Hill Medical Publishing Division.*

Lilly, L et al. Pathophysiology of Heart Disease, Lippincot, Williams and Williams, 1997

Nadas' Pediatric Cardiology 2nd Edition. Philadelphia: Elsevier.

Pocock, Gillian. *Human Physiology* (Third ed.). Oxford University Press

Shabetai R. Constrictive pericarditis. Shabetai R, ed. *The Pericardium*. New York, NY: Grune & Stratton; 1981.

Shabetai R. *Pericardial Disease: etiology, pathophysiology, clinical recognition, and treatment.* New York NY: Churchill Livingstone; 1995. 1024-31

Topol EJ (Ed), Textbook of Cardiovascular Medicine, Lippincott-Raven, Philadelphia 1998.

ARTICLES IN MEDICAL JOURNALS

CASE 2: MITRAL STENOSIS

Ben Farhat M, Ayari M, Maatouk F, et al. Percutaneous balloon versus surgical closed and open mitral commissurotomy: seven-year follow-up results of a randomized trial. *Circulation.* 1998; 97:245.

John S, Bashi VV, Jairaj PS, et al. Closed mitral valvotomy: early results and long-term follow-up of 3724 consecutive patients. *Circulation.* 1983; 68:891.

Khan MN. The relief of mitral stenosis. An historic step in cardiac surgery. *Tex Heart In st J.* 1996; 23:258.

Lau KW, Ding ZP, Hung JS. Percutaneous transvenous mitral commissurotomy versus surgical commissurotomy in the treatment of mitral stenosis. *Clin Cardiol.* 1997; 20:99.

Nishimura RA, Otto CM, Bonow RO, et al. 2014 AHA/ACC guideline for the management of patients with valvular heart disease: a report of the American College of Cardiology/American Heart Association Task Force on Practice Guidelines. *J Am Coll Cardiol.* 2014; 63:

Reyes VP, Raju BS, Wynne J, et al. Percutaneous balloon valvuloplasty compared with open surgical commissurotomy for mitral stenosis. *N Engl J Med.* 1994; 331:961.

Wheeler EO, Wilkins GT, Reynolds TR, et al.. Rheumatic mitral valve disease and tricuspid valve disease. In: *The Practice of Cardiology*, 2nd ed, Eagle KA, Habe E

CASE 3: MITRAL REGURGITATION

Carabello BA, Nolan SP, McGuire LB. Assessment of preoperative left ventricular function in patients with mitral regurgitation: value of the end-systolic wall stress-end-systolic volume ratio. *Circulation.* 1981; 64:1212.

Corin WJ, Monrad ES, Murakami T, et al. The relationship of afterload to ejection performance in chronic mitral regurgitation. *Circulation.* 1987; 76:59.

Corin WJ, Sütsch G, Murakami T, et al. Left ventricular function in chronic mitral regurgitation: preoperative and postoperative comparison. *J Am Coll Cardiol* 1995; 25:113.

Goldfine H, Aurigemma GP, Zile MR, Gaasch WH. Left ventricular length-force-shortening relations before and after surgical correction of chronic mitral regurgitation. *J Am Coll Cardiol.* 1998; 31:180.

Zile MR, Gaasch WH, Carroll JD, Levine HJ. Chronic mitral regurgitation: predictive value of preoperative echocardiographic indexes of left ventricular function and wall stress. *J Am Coll Cardiol.* 1984; 3:235.

CASE 4: ACUTE MITRAL REGURGITATION

Estévez-Loureiro R, Arzamendi D, Freixa X, et al. Percutaneous Mitral Valve Repair for Acute Mitral Regurgitation After an Acute Myocardial Infarction. *J Am Coll Cardiol.* 2015; 66:

Feringa HH, Shaw LJ, Poldermans D, et al. Mitral valve repair and replacement in endocarditis: a systematic review of literature. *Ann Thorac Surg.* 2007; 83:564.

Harshaw CW, Grossman W, Munro AB, McLaurin LP. Reduced systemic vascular resistance as therapy for severe mitral regurgitation of valvular origin. *Ann Intern Med.* 1975; 83:312.

Iung B, Rousseau-Paziaud J, Cormier B, et al. Contemporary results of mitral valve repair for infective endocarditis. *J Am Coll Cardiol.* 2004; 43:386.

Lehmann KG, Francis CK, Dodge HT. Mitral regurgitation in early myocardial infarction. Incidence, clinical detection, and prognostic implications. TIMI Study Group. *Ann Intern Med.* 1992; 117:10.

Piérard LA, Lancellotti P. The role of ischemic mitral regurgitation in the pathogenesis of acute pulmonary edema. *N Engl J Med.* 2004; 351:1627.

Roberts WC, Braunwald E, Morrow AG. Acute severe mitral regurgitation secondary to ruptured chordae tendineae: clinical, hemodynamic, and pathologic considerations. *Circulation.* 1966; 33:58.

Russo A, Suri RM, Grigioni F, et al. Clinical outcome after surgical correction of mitral regurgitation due to papillary muscle rupture. *Circulation.* 2008; 118:1528.

Tcheng JE, Jackman JD Jr, Nelson CL, et al. Outcome of patients sustaining acute ischemic mitral regurgitation during myocardial infarction. *Ann Intern Med.* 1992; 117:18.

CASE 5: TRICUSPID REGURGITATION

Frater R. Tricuspid insufficiency. *J Thorac Cardiovasc Surg.* 2001 Sep. 122(3):427-9.

Gatti G, Maffei G, Lusa AM, Pugliese P. Tricuspid valve repair with the Cosgrove-Edwards annuloplasty system: early clinical and echocardiographic results. *Ann Thorac Surg.* 2001 Sep. 72(3):764-7.

Sarano, M. Pathophysiology of tricuspid regurgitation: quantitative Doppler echocardiographic assessment of respiratory dependence. *Circulation.* 2010 Oct 12. 122(15):1505-13..

Shah PM, Raney AA. Tricuspid valve disease. *Curr Probl Cardiol.* 2008 Feb. 33(2):47-84.

Simula DV, Edwards WD, Tazelaar HD, et al. Surgical pathology of carcinoid heart disease: a study of 139 valves from 75 patients spanning 20 years. *Mayo Clin Proc.* 2002 Feb. 77(2):139-47.

Topilsky Y, Khanna AD, Oh JK, et al. Preoperative factors associated with adverse outcome after tricuspid valve replacement. *Circulation.* 2011 May 10. 123(18):1929-39.

CASE 6: VALVULAR AORTIC STENOSIS

Agarwal A, Kini AS, Attanti S, Lee PC, Ashtiani R, Steinheimer AM, et al. Results of repeat balloon valvuloplasty for treatment of aortic stenosis in patients aged 59 to 104 years. *Am J Cardiol*. 2005 Jan 1. 95(1):43-7.

Cowell SJ, Newby DE, Prescott RJ, et al. A randomized trial of intensive lipid-lowering therapy in calcific aortic stenosis. *N Engl J Med*. 2005 Jun 9. 352(23):2389-97.

Lancellotti P, Magne J, Donal E, et al. Clinical outcome in asymptomatic severe aortic stenosis insights from the new proposed aortic stenosis grading classification. *J Am Coll Cardiol*. 2012 Jan 17. 59(3):235-43. [M

Leon MB, Smith CR, Mack M, et al. Transcatheter aortic-valve implantation for aortic stenosis in patients who cannot undergo surgery. *N Engl J Med*. 2010 Oct 21. 363(17):1597-607.

Mack MJ, Leon MB, Smith CR, et al.; for the PARTNER 1 trial investigators. 5-year outcomes of transcatheter aortic valve replacement or surgical aortic valve replacement for high surgical risk patients with aortic stenosis (PARTNER 1): a randomised controlled trial. *Lancet*. 2015 Jun 20. 385 (9986):2477-84.

Rosenhek R, Zilberszac R, Schemper M, Czerny M, Mundigler G, Graf S, et al. Natural history of very severe aortic stenosis. *Circulation*. 2010 Jan 5. 121(1):151-6.

Smith CR, Leon MB, Mack MJ, et al. Transcatheter versus surgical aortic-valve replacement in high-risk patients. *N Engl J Med*. 2011 Jun 9. 364(23):2187-98.

Stassano P, Di Tommaso L, Monaco M, Iorio F, Pepino P, Spampinato N, et al. Aortic valve replacement: a prospective randomized evaluation of mechanical versus biological valves in patients ages 55 to 70 years. *J Am Coll Cardiol*. 2009 Nov 10. 54(20):1862-8.

Tzemos N, Therrien J, Yip J, Thanassoulis G, Tremblay S, Jamorski MT, et al. Outcomes in adults with bicuspid aortic valves. *JAMA*. 2008 Sep 17. 300(11):1317-25.

Zajarias A, Cribier AG. Outcomes and safety of percutaneous aortic valve replacement. *J Am Coll Cardiol*. 2009 May 19. 53(20):1829-36.

CASE 7: CHRONIC AORTIC REGURGITATION

Bekeredjian R, Grayburn PA. Valvular heart disease: aortic regurgitation. *Circulation*. 2005 Jul 5. 112(1):125-34.

BrauKeane MG, Pyeritz RE. Medical management of Marfan syndrome. *Circulation*. 2008 May 27. 117(21):2802-13.

Maurer G. Aortic regurgitation. *Heart*. 2006 Jul. 92(7):994-1000.

Nishimura RA, Otto CM, Bonow RO, Carabello BA, Erwin JP 3rd, Guyton RA, et al. 2014 AHA/ACC Guideline for the Management of Patients With Valvular Heart Disease: a report of the American College of Cardiology/American Heart Association Task Force on Practice Guidelines. *Circulation*. 2014 Jun 10. 129 (23):e521-643. .

Ortiz JT, Shin DD, Rajamannan NM. Approach to the patient with bicuspid aortic valve and ascending aorta aneurysm. *Curr Treat Options Cardiovasc Med*. 2006 Dec. 8(6):461-7. .

Roberts WC, Vowels TJ, Ko JM. Natural history of adults with congenitally malformed aortic valves (unicuspid or bicuspid). *Medicine (Baltimore)*. 2012 Nov. 91(6):287-308. .

Svensson LG, Adams DH, Bonow RO, et al. Aortic valve and ascending aorta guidelines for management and quality measures. *Ann Thorac Surg*. 2013 Jun. 95 (6 Suppl):S1-66.

CASE 8: ACUTE AORTIC REGURGITATION

Morganroth J, Perloff JK, Zeldis SM. Acute severe aortic regurgitation. Pathophysiology, clinical recognition and management. *Ann Intern Med.* 1977;87:223–232.

CASE 9: ACUTE MYOCARDIAL INFARCTION

Crea F, Pupita G, Galassi AR, et al. Role of adenosine in pathogenesis of anginal pain. *Circulation*. 1990 Jan. 81(1):164-72.

Deedwania PC, Carbajal EV. Silent ischemia during daily life is an independent predictor of mortality in stable angina. *Circulation*. 1990 Mar. 81(3):748-56. e].

Fihn SD, Blankenship JC, Alexander KP, Bittl JA, Byrne JG, Fletcher BJ, et al. 2014 ACC/AHA/AATS/PCNA/SCAI/STS focused update of the guideline for the diagnosis and management of patients with stable ischemic heart disease: a report of the American College of Cardiology/American Heart Association Task Force on Practice Guidelines, and the American Association for Thoracic Surgery, Preventive Cardiovascular Nurses Association, Society for Cardiovascular Angiography and Interventions, and Society of Thoracic Surgeons. *Circulation*. 2014 Nov 4. 130 (19):1749-67.

Hemingway H, Langenberg C, Damant J, Frost C, Pyorala K, Barrett-Connor E. Prevalence of angina in women versus men: a systematic review and meta-analysis of international variations across 31 countries. *Circulation*. 2008 Mar 25. 117(12):1526-36.

Kastrati A, Mehilli J, Pache J, et al. Analysis of 14 trials comparing sirolimus-eluting stents with bare-metal stents. *N Engl J Med.* 2007 Mar 8. 356(10):1030-9

Kugiyama K, Yasue H, Okumura K, et al. Nitric oxide activity is deficient in spasm arteries of patients with coronary spastic angina. *Circulation.* 1996 Aug 1. 94(3):266-71.

Maseri A, Crea F, Kaski JC, Davies G. Mechanisms and significance of cardiac ischemic pain. *Prog Cardiovasc Dis.* 1992 Jul-Aug. 35(1):1-18.

Ridker PM, Manson JE, Gaziano JM, et al. Low-dose aspirin therapy for chronic stable angina. A randomized, placebo-controlled clinical trial. *Ann Intern Med.* 1991 May 15. 114(10):835-9.

Yusuf S, Zhao F, Mehta SR, et al. Effects of clopidogrel in addition to aspirin in patients with acute coronary syndromes without ST-segment elevation. *N Engl J Med.* 2001 Aug 16. 345(7):494-502.

CASE 10: VENTRICULAR ANEURYSM

Brown SL, Gropler RJ, Harris KM (May 1997). "Distinguishing left ventricular aneurysm from pseudoaneurysm. A review of the literature". *Chest.* **111** *(5): 1403–9.* doi:10.1378/chest.111.5.14

Zoffoli G, Mangino D, Venturini A, et al. (February 2009). "Diagnosing left ventricular aneurysm from pseudo-aneurysm: a case report and a review in literature". *J Cardiothorac Surg.* **4** *(1): 11.* .

CASE 11: UNSTABLE ANGINA SELECTED REFERENCES

Amsterdam EA, Wenger NK, Brindis RG, et al. 2014 AHA/ACC Guideline for the Management of Patients with Non-ST-Elevation Acute Coronary Syndromes: a report of the American College of Cardiology/American Heart Association Task Force on Practice Guidelines. *J Am Coll Cardiol*. 2014 Dec 23. 64(24):e139-228.

Anderson JL, Adams CD, Antman EM, et al. 2012 ACCF/AHA focused update incorporated into the ACCF/AHA 2007 guidelines for the management of patients with unstable angina/non-ST-elevation myocardial infarction: a report of the American College of Cardiology Foundation/American Heart Association Task Force on Practice Guidelines. *J Am Coll Cardiol*. 2013 Jun 11. 61(23):e179-347.

Cannon CP, McCabe CH, Stone PH, et al. The electrocardiogram predicts one-year outcome of patients with unstable angina and non-Q wave myocardial infarction: results of the TIMI III Registry ECG Ancillary Study. Thrombolysis in Myocardial Ischemia. *J Am Coll Cardiol*. 1997 Jul. 30(1):133-40.

Jneid H, Anderson JL, Wright RS, et al. 2012 ACCF/AHA focused update of the guideline for the management of patients with unstable angina/non-ST-elevation myocardial infarction (updating the 2007 guideline and replacing the 2011 focused update): a report of the American College of Cardiology Foundation/American Heart Association Task Force on Practice Guidelines. *J Am Coll Cardiol*. 2012 Aug 14. 60(7):645-81.

O'Connor FF, Shields DC, Fitzgerald A, Cannon CP, Braunwald E, Fitzgerald DJ. Genetic variation in glycoprotein IIb/IIIa (GPIIb/IIIa) as a determinant of the responses to an oral GPIIb/

IIIa antagonist in patients with unstable coronary syndromes. *Blood*. 2001 Dec 1. 98(12):3256-60.

Scirica BM, Moliterno DJ, Every NR, et al. Differences between men and women in the management of unstable angina pectoris (The GUARANTEE Registry). The GUARANTEE Investigators. *Am J Cardiol*. 1999 Nov 15. 84(10):1145-50.

Skolnick AH, Alexander KP, Chen AY, et al. Characteristics, management, and outcomes of 5,557 patients age > or =90 years with acute coronary syndromes: results from the CRUSADE Initiative. *J Am Coll Cardiol*. 2007 May 1. 49(17):1790-7.

Soukoulis V, Boden WE, Smith SC Jr, O'Gara PT. Nonantithrombotic medical options in acute coronary syndromes: old agents and new lines on the horizon. *Circ Res*. 2014 Jun 6. 114(12):1944-58

White AJ, Duffy SJ, Walton AS, et al. Matrix metalloproteinase-3 and coronary remodelling: implications for unstable coronary disease. *Cardiovasc Res*. 2007 Sep 1. 75(4):813-20.

Willerson JT. Systemic and local inflammation in patients with unstable atherosclerotic plaques. *Prog Cardiovasc Dis*. 2002 May-Jun. 44(6):469-78.

CASE 12–13: MYOCARDIAL INFARCTION AND HEART BLOCK

Rosen, K. Site of Heart Block in Acute Myocardial Infarction | Circulation 1970 D, Ashkenazy J, Kishon Y. Early and late atrioventricular block in acute inferior myocardial infarction.. American J Cardiology 41-35-198 4

CASE 14: MYOCARDIAL INFARCTION AND CARDIOGENIC SHOCK SELECTED REFERENCES.

Alonso DR, Scheidt S, Post M, Killip T. Pathophysiology of cardiogenic shock. Quantification of myocardial necrosis, clinical, pathologic and electrocardiographic correlations. *Circulation*. 1973 Sep. 48 (3):588-96

Babaev A, Frederick PD, Pasta DJ, Every N, Sichrovsky T, Hochman JS. Trends in management and outcomes of patients with acute myocardial infarction complicated by cardiogenic shock. *JAMA*. 2005 Jul 27. 294(4):448-54.

Beyersdorf F, Buckberg GD, Acar C, et al. Cardiogenic shock after acute coronary occlusion. Pathogenesis, early diagnosis, and treatment. *Thorac Cardiovasc Surg*. 1989 Feb. 37 (1):28-36.

De Backer D, Biston P, Devriendt J, et al, for the SOAP II Investigators. Comparison of dopamine and norepinephrine in the treatment of shock. *N Engl J Med*. 2010 Mar 4. 362 (9):779-89.

Goldberg RJ, Samad NA, Yarzebski J, Gurwitz J, Bigelow C, Gore JM. Temporal trends in cardiogenic shock complicating acute myocardial infarction. *N Engl J Med*. 1999 Apr 15. 340(15):1162-8.

Hasdai D, Califf RM, Thompson TD, Hochman JS, Ohman EM, Pfisterer M, et al. Predictors of cardiogenic shock after thrombolytic therapy for acute myocardial infarction. *J Am Coll Cardiol*. 2000 Jan. 35(1):136-43.

Hochman JS, Sleeper LA, White HD, Dzavik V, Wong SC, Menon V, et al. One-year survival following early revascularization for cardiogenic shock. *JAMA*. 2001 Jan 10. 285(2):190-2.

Jeger RV, Radovanovic D, Hunziker PR, Pfisterer ME, Stauffer JC, Erne P, et al. Ten-year trends in the incidence and treatment of cardiogenic shock. *Ann Intern Med.* 2008 Nov 4. 149(9):618-26.

Kolte D, Khera S, Aronow WS, et al. Trends in incidence, management, and outcomes of cardiogenic shock complicating ST-elevation myocardial infarction in the United States. *J Am Heart Assoc.* 2014 Jan 13. 3 (1):e000590.

Picard MH, Davidoff R, Sleeper LA, and the SHOCK Trial investigators. SHould we emergently revascularize Occluded Coronaries for cardiogenic shocK. Echocardiographic predictors of survival and response to early revascularization in cardiogenic shock. *Circulation.* 2003 Jan 21. 107 (2):279-84.

Reynolds HR, Hochman JS. Cardiogenic shock: current concepts and improving outcomes. *Circulation.* 2008 Feb 5. 117(5):686-97. .

Sanborn TA, Sleeper LA, Bates ER, et al. Impact of thrombolysis, intra-aortic balloon pump counterpulsation, and their combination in cardiogenic shock complicating acute myocardial infarction: a report from the SHOCK Trial Registry. SHould we emergently revascularize Occluded Coronaries for cardiogenic shocK?. *J Am Coll Cardiol.* 2000 Sep. 36(3 Suppl A):1123-9.

Sjauw KD, Engstrom AE, Vis MM, et al. A systematic review and meta-analysis of intra-aortic balloon pump therapy in ST-elevation myocardial infarction: should we change the guidelines?. *Eur Heart J.* 2009 Feb. 30 (4):459-68.

CASE 15: MYOCARDIAL INFARCTION. HYPOTENSION

Bates ER. Revisiting reperfusion therapy in inferior myocardial infarction. *J Am Coll Cardiol.* 1997 Aug. 30(2):334-42.

Birnbaum Y, Wagner GS, Barbash GI, et al. Correlation of angiographic findings and right (V1 to V3) versus left (V4 to V6) precordial ST-segment depression in inferior wall acute myocardial infarction. *Am J Cardiol.* 1999 Jan 15. 83(2):143-8.

Braat SH, Brugada P, den Dulk K, van Ommen V, Wellens HJ. Value of lead V4R for recognition of the infarct coronary artery in acute inferior myocardial infarction. *Am J Cardiol.* 1984 Jun 1. 53(11):1538-41.

Forman MB, Goodin J, Phelan B, Kopelman H, Virmani R. Electrocardiographic changes associated with isolated right ventricular infarction. *J Am Coll Cardiol.* 1984 Sep. 4(3):640-3.

Inglessis I, Shin JT, Lepore JJ, et al. Hemodynamic effects of inhaled nitric oxide in right ventricular myocardial infarction and cardiogenic shock. *J Am Coll Cardiol.* 2004 Aug 18. 44(4):793-8.

Kinn JW, Ajluni SC, Samyn JG, Bates ER, Grines CL, O'Neill W. Rapid hemodynamic improvement after reperfusion during right ventricular infarction. *J Am Coll Cardiol.* 1995 Nov 1. 26(5):1230-4.

Roth A, Miller HI, Kaluski E, et al. Early thrombolytic therapy does not enhance the recovery of the right ventricle in patients with acute inferior myocardial infarction and predominant right ventricular involvement. *Cardiology.* 1990. 77(1):40-9.

Schuler G, Hofmann M, Schwarz F, et al. Effect of successful thrombolytic therapy on right ventricular function in acute inferior wall myocardial infarction. *Am J Cardiol.* 1984 Nov 1. 54(8):951-7.

Zeymer U, Neuhaus KL, Wegscheider K, Tebbe U, Molhoek P, Schroder R. Effects of thrombolytic therapy in acute inferior myocardial infarction with or without right ventricular involvement. HIT-4 Trial Group. Hirudin Improvement of Thrombolysis. *J Am Coll Cardiol.* 1998 Oct. 32(4):876-81.

CASE 16: UNSTABLE ANGINA SELECTED REFERENCES

Braunwald, E. "Unstable Angina : An Etiologic Approach to Management". *Circulation.* **98** (21): 2219–2222.

Braunwald, E; "ACC/AHA guideline update for the management of patients with unstable angina and non-ST segment elevation myocardial infarction-2002: Summary Article: A report of the American College of Cardiology/American Heart Association Task Force on Practice Guidelines (Committee on the Management of Patients with Unstable Angina)". *Circulation.* **106** (14): 1893–1900.

Jneid, H; et al. (2012). "2012 ACCF/AHA focused update of the guideline for the management of patients with unstable angina/non-ST-elevation myocardial infarction (updating the 2007 guideline and replacing the 2011 focused update): A report of the American College of Cardiology Foundation/American Heart Association Task Force on Practice Guidelines". *Journal of the American College of Cardiology.* **60** (7): 645–81.

Wiviott, S. D.; Braunwald, E. "Unstable Angina and Non–ST-Segment Elevation Myocardial Infarction: Part I. Initial

Evaluation and Management, and Hospital Care". *American Family Physician*. **70** (3): 525–32.

CASE: ORTHOSTATIC HYPOTENSION

Sim, M; Hudon, R (1979). "Acute intermittent porphyria associated with postural hypotension". *Canadian Medical Association Journal*. **121** (7): 845–6. PMC 1704473

Jiang, Wei; Davidson, Jonathan R.T (2005). "Antidepressant therapy in patients with ischemic heart disease". *American Heart Journal*. **150** (5): 871–81. doi:10.1016/j.ahj.2005.01.041. .

Delini-Stula, A; Baier, D; Kohnen, R; Laux, G; Philipp, M; Scholz, H.-J (2007). "Undesirable Blood Pressure Changes Under Naturalistic Treatment with Moclobemide, a Reversible MAO-A Inhibitor - Results of the Drug Utilization Observation Studies". *Pharmacopsychiatry*. **32** (2): 61–7. doi:10.1055/s-2007-979193.

Jones, Reese T (2002). "Cardiovascular System Effects of Marijuana". *The Journal of Clinical Pharmacology*. **42** (11 Suppl): 58S–63S. doi:10.1002/j.1552-4604.2002.tb06004.x.

Narkiewicz, K; Cooley, R. L; Somers, V. K (2000). "Alcohol potentiates orthostatic hypotension : Implications for alcohol-related syncope". *Circulation*. **101** (4): 398–402. PMID 10653831.

Moya, A; Sutton, R; Ammirati, F; Blanc, J.-J; Brignole, M; Dahm, J. B; Deharo, J.-C; Gajek, J; Gjesdal, K; Krahn, A; Massin, M; Pepi, M; Pezawas, T; Granell, R. R; Sarasin, F; Ungar, A; Van Dijk, J. G; Walma, E. P; Wieling, W; Abe, H; Benditt, D. G; Decker, W. W; Grubb, B. P; Kaufmann, H; Morillo, C; Olshansky, B; Parry, S. W; Sheldon, R; Shen, W. K; et al. (2009). "Guidelines for the diagnosis and management of syncope (version 2009): The Task Force for the Diagnosis and Management of Syncope of the European Society of Cardiology (ESC)". *European Heart Journal.* **30** (21): 2631–71.

Izcovich, A; Gonzalez Malla, C; Manzotti, M; Catalano, H. N; Guyatt, G (2014). "Midodrine for orthostatic hypotension and recurrent reflex syncope: A systematic review". *Neurology.* **83** (13): 117. .

Logan, Ian C; Witham, Miles D (2012). "Efficacy of treatments for orthostatic hypotension: A systematic review". *Age and Ageing.* **41** (5): 587–94. doi:10.1093/ageing/afs061..

Romero-Ortuno, Roman; Cogan, Lisa; Foran, Tim; Kenny, Rose Anne; Fan, Chie Wei (2011). "Continuous Noninvasive Orthostatic Blood Pressure Measurements and Their Relationship with Orthostatic Intolerance, Falls, and Frailty in Older People" (PDF). *Journal of the American Geriatrics Society.* **59** (4): 655–65. doi:10.1111/j.1532-5415.2011.03352.x.

Ricci, Fabrizio; Fedorowski, Artur; Radico, Francesco; Romanello, Mattia; Tatasciore, Alfonso; Di Nicola, Marta; Zimarino, Marco; De Caterina, Raffaele (2015). "Cardiovascular morbidity and mortality related to orthostatic hypotension: A meta-analysis of prospective observational studies". *European Heart Journal.* **36** (25): 1609–17. doi:10.1093/eurheartj/ehv093.

Rawlings, Andreea; et al. (March 2017). Orthostatic Hypotension is Associated With 20-year Cognitive Decline and Incident Dementia: the Atherosclerosis Risk in Communities (ARIC) Study (PDF). Epidemiology and Prevention / Lifestyle and Cardiometabolic Health 2017 Scientific Sessions. Portland, Oregon.

CASE: MI and VENTRICULAR TACHYCARDIA

Aliot EM, Stevenson WG, Almendral-Garrote JM, et al.. "EHRA/HRS Expert Consensus on Catheter Ablation of Ventricular Arrhythmias: developed in a partnership with the European Heart Rhythm Association (EHRA), a Registered Branch of the European Society of Cardiology (ESC), and the Heart Rhythm Society (HRS); in collaboration with the American College of Cardiology (ACC) and the American Heart Association (AHA)".

Brugada P, Brugada J, Mont L, Smeets J, Andries EW. "A new approach to the differential diagnosis of a regular tachycardia with a wide QRS complex". *Circulation.* **83** (5): 1649–59.

deSouza, IS; Martindale, JL; Sinert, R . "Antidysrhythmic drug therapy for the termination of stable, monomorphic ventricular tachycardia: a systematic review.". *Emergency medicine journal : EMJ.* **32** (2): 161–167.

John RM, Tedrow UB, Koplan BA, et al. "Ventricular arrhythmias and sudden cardiac death". *Lancet.* **380** (9852): 1520–9.

Stewart RB, Bardy GH, Greene HL. "Wide complex tachycardia: misdiagnosis and outcome after emergent therapy". *Annals of Internal Medicine.* **104** (6): 766–71.

Wellens HJ, Bär FW, Lie KI. "The value of the electrocardiogram in the differential diagnosis of a tachycardia with a widened QRS complex". *The American Journal of Medicine.* **64** (1): 27–33.

CASE 17: DILATED CARDIOMYOPATHY

Barbaro G. Cardiovascular manifestations of HIV infection. *Circulation.* 2002 Sep 10. 106 (11):1420-5.

Canter CE, Simpson KE. Diagnosis and treatment of myocarditis in children in the current era. *Circulation*. 2014 Jan 7. 129 (1):115-28. .

Kayvanpour, Elham; Sedaghat-Hamedani, Farbod; Amr, Ali; Lai, Alan; Haas, Jaan; Holzer, Daniel B.; Frese, Karen S.; Keller, Andreas; Jensen, Katrin; Katus, Hugo A.; Meder, Benjamin (2016-08-30). "Genotype-phenotype associations in dilated cardiomyopathy: meta-analysis on more than 8000 individuals". *Clinical Research in Cardiology*. .

Likoff MJ, Chandler SL, Kay HR. Clinical determinants of mortality in chronic congestive heart failure secondary to idiopathic dilated or to ischemic cardiomyopathy. *Am J Cardiol*. 1987 Mar 1. 59 (6):634-8.

Martino TA, Liu P, Sole MJ. "Viral infection and the pathogenesis of dilated cardiomyopathy". *Circ Res*. **74** (2): 182–8.

Mason JW, O'Connell JB, Herskowitz A, et al. A clinical trial of immunosuppressive therapy for myocarditis. The Myocarditis Treatment Trial Investigators. *N Engl J Med*. 1995 Aug 3. 333(5):269-75. .

McNamara DM, Holubkov R, Starling RC, et al. Controlled trial of intravenous immune globulin in recent-onset dilated cardiomyopathy. *Circulation*. 2001 May 8. 103 (18):2254-9.

Mouhaffel AH, Madu EC, Satmary WA, Fraker TD Jr. Cardiovascular complications of cocaine. *Chest*. 1995 May. 107 (5):1426-34. .

Nikolic G, Marriott HJ. "Left bundle branch block with right axis deviation: a marker of congestive cardiomyopathy". *J Electrocardiol*. **18** (4): 395–404.

Ross J. "Dilated cardiomyopathy: concepts derived from gene deficient and transgenic animal models". *Circ J.* **66** (3): 219–24. :

Sekhri V, Sanal S, Delorenzo LJ, Aronow WS, Maguire GP. Cardiac sarcoidosis: a comprehensive review. *Arch Med Sci.* 2011 Aug. 7 (4):546-54.

Sliwa K, Fett J, Elkayam U. Peripartum cardiomyopathy. *Lancet.* 2006 Aug 19. 368 (9536):687-93.

van Spaendonck-Zwarts KY, van Tintelen JP, van Veldhuisen DJ, van der Werf R, Jongbloed JD, Paulus WJ, et al. Peripartum cardiomyopathy as a part of familial dilated cardiomyopathy. *Circulation.* 2010 May 25. 121(20):2169-75.

Virani SS, Khan AN, Mendoza CE, Ferreira AC, de Marchena E. Takotsubo cardiomyopathy, or broken-heart syndrome. *Tex Heart Inst J.* 2007. 34 (1):76-9

CASE 18: DIASTOLIC HEART FAILURE—SELECTED REFERENCES

Topol,E; Robert M. Califf (2007). *Textbook of cardiovascular medicine.* Lippincott Williams & Wilkins. pp. 420.

Articles in Medical Journals

Bhatia RS, Tu JV, Lee DS, et al. (July 2006). "Outcome of heart failure with preserved ejection fraction in a population-based study". *N. Engl. J. Med.* **355** (3): 260.

Germing, A.; Gotzmann, M.; Schikowski, T.; Vierkötter, A.; Ranft, U.; Krämer, U.; Mügge, A. (2011). "High frequency of diastolic dysfunction in a population-based cohort of elderly women - but poor association with the symptom dyspnea". *BMC Geriatrics*. **11**: 71.

Owan TE, Hodge DO, Herges RM, Jacobsen SJ, Roger VL, Redfield MM (July 2006). "Trends in prevalence and outcome of heart failure with preserved ejection fraction". *N. Engl. J. Med.* **355** (3): 251–59. .

CASE 19: RESTRICTIVE CARDIOMYOPATHY—SELECTED REFERENCES

Artz, Gregory; Wynne, Joshua. "Restrictive Cardiomyopathy". Current Treatment Options in Cardiovascular Medicine. **2** (5): 431–438.

Gertz, Morie A.; Falk, Rodney H.; Skinner, Martha; Cohen, Alan S.; Kyle, Robert A.. "Worsening of congestive heart failure in amyloid heart disease treated by calcium channel-blocking agents". *American Journal of Cardiology*. **55** (13): 1645.

Hancock, EW. "Differential diagnosis of restrictive cardiomyopathy and constrictive pericarditis". *Heart (British Cardiac Society)*. **86** (3): 343–9.

Pollak, A; Falk, R H. "Left ventricular systolic dysfunction precipitated by verapamil in cardiac amyloidosis.". *Chest*. **104** (2): 618–620.

Stöllberger, C.; Finsterer, J. "Extracardiac medical and neuromuscular implications in restrictive cardiomyopathy". *Clinical Cardiology*. **30** (8): 375–380.

CASE 20: OBSTRUCTIVE CARDIOMYOPATHY—SELECTED REFERENCES

Galve E, Sambola A, Saldaña G, Quispe I, Nieto E, Diaz A, et al. Late benefits of dual- Gersh BJ, Maron BJ, Bonow RO, et al, for the American College of Cardiology Foundation/American Heart Association Task Force on Practice Guidelines. 2011 ACCF/AHA guideline for the diagnosis and treatment of hypertrophic cardiomyopathy: a report of the American College of Cardiology Foundation/American Heart Association Task Force on Practice Guidelines. Developed in collaboration with the American Association for Thoracic Surgery, American Society of Echocardiography, American Society of Nuclear Cardiology, Heart Failure Society of America, Heart Rhythm Society, Society for Cardiovascular Angiography and Interventions, and Society of Tho... *J Am Coll Cardiol*. 2011 Dec 13. 58 (25):e212-60.

Jensen MK, Prinz C, Horstkotte D, van Buuren F, Bitter T, Faber L, et al. Alcohol septal ablation in patients with hypertrophic obstructive cardiomyopathy: low incidence of sudden cardiac death and reduced risk profile. *Heart*. 2013 Jul. 99(14):1012-7.

Maron BJ, Gardin JM, Flack JM, et al. Prevalence of hypertrophic cardiomyopathy in a general population of young adults. Echocardiographic analysis of 4111 subjects in the CARDIA Study. Coronary Artery Risk Development in (Young) Adults. *Circulation*. 1995 Aug 15. 92(4):785-9.

Maron BJ, Roberts WC, Epstein SE. Sudden death in hypertrophic cardiomyopathy: a profile of 78 patients. *Circulation*. 1982 Jun. 65(7):1388-94. .

Maron BJ. Hypertrophic cardiomyopathy: a systematic review. *JAMA*. 2002 Mar 13. 287(10):1308-20.

Soor GS, Luk A, Ahn E, Abraham JR, Woo A, Ralph-Edwards A, et al. Hypertrophic cardiomyopathy: current understanding and treatment objectives. *J Clin Pathol*. 2009 Mar. 62(3):226-35.

Van Driest SL, Ackerman MJ, Ommen SR, Shakur R, Will ML, Nishimura RA, et Maron BJ, McKenna WJ, Danielson GK, Kappenberger LJ, Kuhn HJ, Seidman CE, et al. American College of Cardiology/European Society of Cardiology clinical expert consensus document on hypertrophic cardiomyopathy. A report of the American College of Cardiology Foundation Task Force on Clinical Expert Consensus Documents and the European Society of Cardiology Committee for Practice Guidelines. *J Am Coll Cardiol*. 2003 Nov 5. 42(9):1687-713.

Vriesendorp PA, Schinkel AF, Soliman OI, et al. Long-term benefit of myectomy and anterior mitral leaflet extension in obstructive hypertrophic cardiomyopathy. *Am J Cardiol*. 2015 Mar 1. 115 (5):670-5.

CASE 20: CARDIAC TAMPONADE—SELECTED REFERENCES

Cornily JC, Pennec PY, Castellant P, Bezon E, Le Gal G, Gilard M, et al. Cardiac tamponade in medical patients: a 10-year follow-up survey. *Cardiology*. 2008. 111(3):197-201.

Holmes DR Jr, Nishimura R, Fountain R, et al. Iatrogenic pericardial effusion and tamponade in the percutaneous intracardiac intervention era. *JACC Cardiovasc Interv*. 2009 Aug. 2(8):705-17.

Miralda G, Soler-Soler J. Low-pressure cardiac tamponade: clinical and hemodynamic profile. *Circulation*. 2006 Aug 29. 114(9):945-52..

Reddy PS, Curtiss EI, Uretsky BF. Spectrum of hemodynamic changes in cardiac tamponade. *Am J Cardiol*. 1990 Dec 15. 66(20):1487-91.

Sagrista-Sauleda J, Angel J, Sambola A, Permanyer-Miralda G. Hemodynamic effects of volume expansion in patients with cardiac tamponade. *Circulation*. 2008 Mar 25. 117(12):1545-9.

Stone MK, Bauch TD, Rubal BJ. Respiratory changes in the pulse-oximetry waveform associated with pericardial tamponade. *Clin Cardiol*. 2006 Sep. 29(9):411-4.

You SC, Shim CY, Hong GR, et al. Incidence, predictors, and clinical outcomes of postoperative cardiac tamponade in patients undergoing heart valve surgery. *PLoS One*. 2016 Nov 17. 11 (11):e0165754.

CASE 21: CONSTRICTIVE PERICARDITIS—SELECTED REFERENCES

Bertog SC, Thambidorai SK, Parakh K, et al. Constrictive pericarditis: etiology and cause-specific survival after pericardiectomy. *J Am Coll Cardiol*. 2004 Apr 21. 43(8):1445-52.

Brockington GM, Zebede J, Pandian NG. Constrictive pericarditis. *Cardiol Clin*. 1990 Nov. 8(4):645-61.

Clare GC, Troughton RW. Management of constrictive pericarditis in the 21st century. *Curr Treat Options Cardiovasc Med*. 2007 Dec. 9(6):436-42..

Imazio M, Brucato A, Maestroni S, et al. Risk of constrictive pericarditis after acute pericarditis. *Circulation*. 2011 Sep 13. 124(11):1270-5..

Leya FS, Arab D, Joyal D, et al. The efficacy of brain natriuretic peptide levels in differentiating constrictive pericarditis from restrictive cardiomyopathy. *J Am Coll Cardiol*. 2005 Jun 7. 45(11):1900-2

Ling LH, Oh JK, Schaff HV, et al. Constrictive pericarditis in the modern era: evolving clinical spectrum and impact on outcome after pericardiectomy. *Circulation*. 1999 Sep 28. 100(13):1380-6..

Tuna IC, Danielson GK. Surgical management of pericardial diseases. *Cardiol Clin*. 1990 Nov. 8(4):683-96.

Veress G, Feng D, Oh JK. Echocardiography in pericardial diseases: new developments Use of magnetic resonance imaging in assessment of constrictive pericarditis: a Moroccan center experience. *Int Arch Med*. 2011 Oct 19. 4(1):36. *Heart Fail Rev*. 2012 Jul 1.

Yazdani K, Maraj S, Amanullah AM. Differentiating constrictive pericarditis from restrictive cardiomyopathy. *Rev Cardiovasc Med*. 2005. 6(2):61-71.

CASE 22: COMPLETE HEART BLOCK

Bestetti RB, Cury PM, Theodoropoulos TA, Villafanha D. Trypanosoma cruzi myocardial infection reactivation presenting as complete atrioventricular block in a Chagas' heart transplant recipient. *Cardiovasc Pathol*. 2004 Nov-Dec. 13(6):323-6.

Bestetti RB, Cury PM, Theodoropoulos TA, Villafanha D. Trypanosoma cruzi myocardial infection reactivation presenting as complete atrioventricular block in a Chagas' heart transplant recipient. *Cardiovasc Pathol*. 2004 Nov-Dec. 13(6):323-6.

Kojic EM, Hardarson T, Sigfusson N, Sigvaldason H. The prevalence and prognosis of third-degree atrioventricular conduction block: the Reykjavik study. *J Intern Med*. 1999 Jul. 246(1):81-6..

Narula OS, Scherlag BJ, Javier RP, Hildner FJ, Samet P. Analysis of the A-V conduction defect in complete heart block utilizing His bundle electrograms. *Circulation*. 1970 Mar. 41(3):437-48.

Narula OS, Scherlag BJ, Javier RP, Hildner FJ, Samet P. Analysis of the A-V conduction defect in complete heart block utilizing His bundle electrograms. *Circulation*. 1970 Mar. 41(3):437-48.

Rosen KM, Dhingra RC, Loeb HS, Rahimtoola SH. Chronic heart block in adults. Clinical and electrophysiological observations. *Arch Intern Med*. 1973 May. 131(5):663-72.

Rosen KM, Dhingra RC, Loeb HS, Rahimtoola SH. Chronic heart block in adults. Clinical and electrophysiological observations. *Arch Intern Med*. 1973 May. 131(5):663-72.

Tracy CM, Epstein AE, Darbar D, Dimarco JP, Dunbar SB, Estes NA 3rd, et al. 2012 ACCF/AHA/HRS focused update of the 2008 guidelines for device-based therapy of cardiac rhythm abnormalities: a report of the American College of Cardiology Foundation/American Heart Association Task Force on Practice Guidelines. *J Am Coll Cardiol*. 2012 Oct 2. 60(14):1297-313.

CASE 23: BRADYARRHYTHMIAS SICK SINUS SYNDROME

Adán V, Crown LA (April 2003). "Diagnosis and treatment of sick sinus syndrome". *Am Fam Physician*. 67 (8): 1725–32.

Keller KB, Lemberg L (March 2006). "The sick sinus syndrome". *Am. J. Crit. Care.* 15 (2): 226–9.

Drago F, Silvetti MS, Grutter G, De Santis A (July 2006). "Long term management of atrial arrhythmias in young patients with sick sinus syndrome undergoing early operation to correct congenital heart disease". *Europace.* 8 (7): 488–94.

Dobrzynski H, Boyett MR, Anderson RH (April 2007). "New insights into pacemaker activity: promoting understanding of sick sinus syndrome". *Circulation.* 115 (14): 1921–32.

Semelka, M; Gera, J; Usman, S (May 2013). "Sick sinus syndrome: a review". *American Family Physician (Review).* 87 (10): 691-6.

CASE 24: MOBITZ 1

Coumbe AG, Naksuk N, Newell MC, Somasundaram PE, Benditt DG, Adabag S. Long-term follow-up of older patients with Mobitz type I second degree atrioventricular block. *Heart.* 2013 Mar. 99(5):334-8..

Hsu YJ, Lin YF, Chau T, et al. Electrocardiographic manifestations in patients with thyrotoxic periodic paralysis. *Am J Med Sci.* 2003 Sep. 326(3):128-32.

Lev M. Anatomic basis for atrioventricular block. *Am J Med.* 1964 Nov. 37:742-8.

Strasberg B, Amat-Y-Leon F, Dhingra RC, et al. Natural history of chronic second-degree atrioventricular nodal block. *Circulation.* 1981 May. 63(5):1043-9. .

Thanopoulos BD, Rigby ML. Outcome of transcatheter closure of muscular ventricular septal defects with the Amplatzer ventricular septal defect occluder. *Heart.* 2005 Apr. 91(4):513-6.

Van Herendael B, Van Herendael H, De Raedt H. Second-degree atrioventricular block as the first sign of sarcoidosis in a previously asymptomatic patient. *Acta Cardiol.* 2007 Jun. 62(3):299-301.

CASE 26: SUPRAVENTRICULAR TACHYCARDIA

Akhtar M, Jazayeri MR, Sra J, Blanck Z, Deshpande S, Dhala A. Atrioventricular nodal reentry. Clinical, electrophysiological, and therapeutic considerations. *Circulation.* 1993 Jul. 88(1):282-95.
Wissner E, Stevenson WG, Kuck KH (June 2012). "Catheter ablation of ventricular tachycardia in ischaemic and non-ischaemic cardiomyopathy: where are we today? A clinical review". European Heart Journal. 33 (12): 1440–50.

Basta M, Klein GJ, Yee R, Krahn A, Lee J. Current role of pharmacologic therapy for patients with paroxysmal supraventricular tachycardia. *Cardiol Clin.* 1997 Nov. 15(4):587-97.

Denes P, Wu D, Dhingra RC, Chuquimia R, Rosen KM. Demonstration of dual A-V nodal pathways in patients with paroxysmal supraventricular tachycardia. *Circulation.* 1973 Sep. 48(3):549-55.

Ganz LI, Friedman PL. Supraventricular tachycardia. *N Engl J Med.* 1995 Jan 19. 332(3):162-73.

Josephson ME, Kastor JA. Supraventricular tachycardia: mechanisms and management. *Ann Intern Med.* 1977 Sep. 87(3):346-58.

Klein GJ, Sharma AD, Yee R, Guiraudon GM. Classification of supraventricular tachycardias. *Am J Cardiol.* 1987 Aug 31. 60(6):27D-31D..

Lesh MD, Van Hare GF, Epstein LM, et al. Radiofrequency catheter ablation of atrial arrhythmias. Results and mechanisms. *Circulation.* 1994 Mar. 89(3):1074-89. [Medline].

Rosen KM, Mehta A, Miller RA. Demonstration of dual atrioventricular nodal pathways in man. *Am J Cardiol.* 1974 Feb. 33(2):291-4.

CASE 27: WPW—SELECTED REFERENCES

Beckman NL, Lamb LE. The Wolff-Parkinson-White electrocardiogram; follow-up study of five to twenty-eight years. *N Engl J Med.* 1968;278:492.

Brembilla-Perrot B, Ghawi R. Electrophysiological characteristics of asymptomatic Wolff-Parkinson-White syndrome. *Eur Heart J.* 1993;14:511–515

Brembilla-Perrot B, Holban I, Houriez P, et al. Influence of age on the potential risk of sudden death in asymptomatic Wolff-Parkinson-White syndrome. *PACE.* 2001;24:1514–1518

Fitzsimmons PJ, Mc Whirter PD, Peterson DW, et al. The natural history of Wolff-Parkinson-White syndrome in 228 military aviators : a long-term follow-up of 22 years. *Am Heart J.* 2001;142:530–536.

Warin JF, Haissaguerre M, Lemetayer P, et al. Catheter ablation of accessory pathways with a direct approach. Results in 35 patients. *Circulation.* 1988;78:800–815

Wellens HJJ, Bar FW, Dassen WR, et al. Effects of drugs in the Wolff Parkinson White syndrome . Importance of initial length of effective refractory period in the accessory pathway. *Am J Cardiol.* 1980;46:665–669.

CASE 27–28: ATRIAL FIBRILLATION AND FLUTTER

Abi-Mansour P, Carberry PA, McCowan RJ, Henthorn RW, Dunn GH, Perry KT. Conversion efficacy and safety of repeated doses of ibutilide in patients with atrial flutter and atrial fibrillation. Study Investigators. *Am Heart J.* 1998 Oct. 136(4 Pt 1):632-42.

Allessie M, Ausma J, Schotten U. Electrical, contractile and structural remodeling during atrial fibrillation. *Cardiovasc Res.* 2002 May. 54 (2):230-46.

Berger M, Schweitzer P. Timing of thromboembolic events after electrical cardioversion of atrial fibrillation or flutter: a retrospective analysis. *Am J Cardiol.* 1998 Dec 15. 82(12):1545-7,

Biblo LA, Yuan Z, Quan KJ, Mackall JA, Rimm AA. Risk of stroke in patients with atrial flutter. *Am J Cardiol.* 2001 Feb 1. 87(3):346-9, A9. ..

Burstein B, Nattel S. Atrial fibrosis: mechanisms and clinical relevance in atrial fibrillation. *J Am Coll Cardiol.* 2008 Feb 26. 51 (8):802-9..

Everett BM, Cook NR, Conen D, Chasman DI, Ridker PM, Albert CM. Novel genetic markers improve measures of atrial fibrillation risk prediction. *Eur Heart J.* 2013 Aug. 34 (29):2243-51. .

Fox CS, Parise H, D'Agostino RB Sr, et al. Parental atrial fibrillation as a risk factor for atrial fibrillation in offspring. *JAMA*. 2004 Jun 16. 291 (23):2851-5.

Frustaci A, Chimenti C, Bellocci F, Morgante E, Russo MA, Maseri A. Histological substrate of atrial biopsies in patients with lone atrial fibrillation. *Circulation*. 1997 Aug 19. 96 (4):1180-4.

Granada J, Uribe W, Chyou PH, Maassen K, Vierkant R, Smith PN, et al. Incidence and predictors of atrial flutter in the general population. *J Am Coll Cardiol*. 2000 Dec. 36(7):2242-6.

January CT, Wann LS, Alpert JS, et al, for the American College of Cardiology/American Heart Association Task Force on Practice Guidelines. 2014 AHA/ACC/HRS guideline for the management of patients with atrial fibrillation: a report of the American College of Cardiology/American Heart Association Task Force on Practice Guidelines and the Heart Rhythm Society. *J Am Coll Cardiol*. 2014 Dec 2. 64 (21):e1-76.

Hagens VE, Ranchor AV, Van Sonderen E, et al, for the RACE Study Group. Effect of rate or rhythm control on quality of life in persistent atrial fibrillation. Results from the Rate Control Versus Electrical Cardioversion (RACE) Study. *J Am Coll Cardiol*. 2004 Jan 21. 43 (2):241-7.

Holmes DR Jr, Doshi SK, Kar S, et al. Left atrial appendage closure as an alternative to warfarin for stroke prevention in atrial fibrillation: a patient-level meta-analysis. *J Am Coll Cardiol*. 2015 Jun 23. 65 (24):2614-23.

Hoyt H, Bhonsale A, Chilukuri K, et al. Complications arising from catheter ablation of atrial fibrillation: temporal trends and predictors. *Heart Rhythm*. 2011 Dec. 8 (12):1869-74.

Kannel WB, Wolf PA, Benjamin EJ, Levy D. Prevalence, incidence, prognosis, and predisposing conditions for atrial fibrillation: population-based estimates. *Am J Cardiol.* 1998 Oct 16. 82 (8A):2N-9N.

McNamara RL, Tamariz LJ, Segal JB, Bass EB. Management of atrial fibrillation: review of the evidence for the role of pharmacologic therapy, electrical cardioversion, and echocardiography. *Ann Intern Med.* 2003 Dec 16. 139 (12):1018-33.

Pappone C, Rosanio S, Oreto G, et al. Circumferential radiofrequency ablation of pulmonary vein ostia: a new anatomic approach for curing atrial fibrillation. *Circulation.* 2000 Nov 21. 102 (21):2619-28. .

Roux JF, Zado E, Callans DJ, et al. Antiarrhythmics After Ablation of Atrial Fibrillation (5A Study). *Circulation.* 2009 Sep 22. 120 (12):1036-40. .

Stollberger C, Chnupa P, Abzieher C, et al. Mortality and rate of stroke or embolism in atrial fibrillation during long-term follow-up in the Embolism in Left Atrial Thrombi (ELAT) Study. *Clin Cardiol.* 2004 Jan. 27 (1):40-6. [Medline].

Winkle RA, Mead RH, Engel G, Patrawala RA. Long-term results of atrial fibrillation ablation: the importance of all initial ablation failures undergoing a repeat ablation. *Am Heart J.* 2011 Jul. 162 (1):193-200. .

CASE 29: LONG QT SYNDROME

Compton SJ, Lux RL, Ramsey MR, et al. (1996). "Genetically defined therapy of inherited long-QT syndrome. Correction of abnormal repolarization by potassium". *Circulation.* **94** (5): 1018–22.

Ellinor PT, Milan DJ, MacRae CA; Milan; MacRae (2003). "Risk stratification in the long-QT syndrome". *N. Engl. J. Med.* **349** (9): 908–9.

Jervell A, Lange-Nielsen F; Lange-Nielsen (July 1957). "Congenital deaf-mutism, functional heart disease with prolongation of the Q-T interval and sudden death". *Am. Heart J.* **54** (1): 59–68.

Levine E, Rosero SZ, Budzikowski AS, Moss AJ, Zareba W, Daubert JP; Rosero; Budzikowski; Moss; Zareba; Daubert (August 2008). "Congenital long QT syndrome: considerations for primary care physicians". *Cleve Clin J Med.* **75** (8): 591–600

Moric-Janiszewska E, Markiewicz-Łoskot G, Loskot M, Weglarz L, Hollek A, Szydlowski L; Markiewicz-Łoskot; Łoskot; Weglarz; Hollek; Szydłowski (2007). "Challenges of diagnosis of long-QT syndrome in children". *Pacing Clin Electrophysiol.* **30** (9): 1168–1170.

Schwartz PJ, Moss AJ, Vincent GM, Crampton RS; Moss; Vincent; Crampton (1993). "Diagnostic criteria for the long QT syndrome. An update". *Circulation.* **88** (2): 782–4.

Wang F, Liu J, Hong L, et al. (2013). "The phenotype characteristics of type 13 long QT syndrome with mutation in KCNJ5 (Kir3.4-G387R).". *Heart Rhythm.* **10** (10): 1500–6.

CASE 28: VENTRICULAR SEPTAL DEFECT

Fu, YC (February 2011). "Transcatheter device closure of muscular ventricular septal defect.". *Pediatrics and neonatology.* **52** (1): 3–4. .

Hoffman, JI; Kaplan, S (2002). "The incidence of congenital heart disease". *Journal of the American College of Cardiology.* **39** (12): 1890–900. .

Roguin, Nathan; Du, Zhong-Dong; Barak, Mila; Nasser, Nadim; Hershkowitz, Sylvia; Milgram, Elliot . "High prevalence of muscular ventricular septal defect in neonates". *Journal of the American College of Cardiology.* **26** (6): 1545–154

CASE 29: ATRIAL SEPTAL DEFECT

Bedford DE. The anatomical types of atrial septal defect. Their incidence and clinical diagnosis. *Am J Cardiol.* 1960 Sep. 6:568-74.

Cherian G, Uthaman CB, Durairaj M, et al. Pulmonary hypertension in isolated secundum atrial septal defect: high frequency in young patients. *Am Heart J.* 1983 Jun. 105(6):952-7. .

Dutty S, Hazeem AA, Brown K, et al. Long-term (5- to 20-year) outcomes after transcatheter or surgical treatment of hemodynamically significant isolated secundum atrial septal defect. *Am J Cardiol.* 2012 May 1. 109(9):1348-52.

Fischer G, Stieh J, Uebing A, Hoffmann U, Morf G, Kramer HH. Experience with transcatheter closure of secundum atrial septal defects using the Amplatzer septal occluder: a single centre study in 236 consecutive patients. *Heart.* 2003 Feb. 89(2):199-204.

Isselbacher KJ, Braunwald E, Wilson JD. Atrial septal defect. In: Isselbacher KJ, ed. *Harrison's Principles of Internal Medicine.* 13th ed. New York, NY: McGraw-Hill; 1994. 1041.

Krumsdorf U, Ostermayer S, Billinger K, et al. Incidence and clinical course of thrombus formation on atrial septal defect and patient foramen ovale closure devices in 1,000 consecutive patients. *J Am Coll Cardiol*. 2004 Jan 21. 43(2):302-9.

Marelli AJ, Moodie DS, Topol EJ. Adult congenital heart disease. *Textbook of Cardiovascular Medicine*. Philadelphia, Pa: Lippincott-Raven; 1998. 775-9..

Sealy WC, Farmer JC, Young Jr WG, et al. Atrial dysrhythmia and atrialsecundum defects. *J Thorac Cardiovasc Surg*. 1969 Feb. 57(2):245-50.

Stark J. Secundum atrial septal defect. *Surgery for Congenital Heart Defects*. New York, NY: Gru

Warnes CA, Williams RG, Bashore TM, et al. ACC/AHA 2008 guidelines for the management of adults with congenital heart disease: executive summary: a report of the American College of Cardiology/American Heart Association Task Force on Practice Guidelines (writing committee to develop guidelines for the management of adults with congenital heart disease). *Circulation*. 2008 Dec 2. 118(23):2395-451.

Warnes CA. The adult with congenital heart disease: born to be bad?. *J Am Coll Cardiol*. 2005 Jul 5. 46(1):1-8.

Webb G, Gatzoulis MA. Atrial septal defects in the adult: recent progress and overview. *Circulation*. 2006 Oct 10. 114(15):1645-53.

CASE 30: PATENT DUCTUS ARTERIOSUS

Castaneda A. Congenital heart disease: a surgical-historical perspective. *Ann Thorac Surg*. 2005 Jun. 79(6):S2217-20.

Chen Z, Chen L, Wu L. Transcatheter amplatzer occlusion and surgical closure of patent ductus arteriosus: comparison of effectiveness and costs in a low-income country. *Pediatr Cardiol.* 2009 Aug. 30(6):781-5.

Lin CC, Hsieh KS, Huang TC, Weng KP. Closure of large patent ductus arteriosus in infants. *Am J Cardiol.* 2009 Mar 15. 103(6):857-61. .

Nuntnarumit P, Chongkongkiat P, Khositseth A. N-terminal-pro-brain natriuretic peptide: a guide for early targeted indomethacin therapy for patent ductus arteriosus in preterm Infants. *Acta Paediatr.* 2011 Sep. 100(9):1217-21.

Rapacciuolo A, Losi MA, Borgia F, et al. Transcatheter closure of patent ductus arteriosus reverses left ventricular dysfunction in a septuagenarian. *J Cardiovasc Med (Hagerstown).* 2009 Apr. 10(4):344-8.

Schneider DJ, Moore JW. Patent ductus arteriosus. *Circulation.* 2006 Oct 24. 114(17):1873-82.

Takami T, Yoda H, Kawakami T, et al. Usefulness of indomethacin for patent ductus arteriosus in full-term infants. *Pediatr Cardiol.* 2007 Jan-Feb. 28(1):46-50.

CASE 31: VENTRICULAR SEPTAL DEFECT—PULMONARY HYPERTENSION

Bando K, Vijayaraghavan P, Turrentine MW, et al. Dynamic changes of endothelin-1, nitric oxide, and cyclic GMP in patients with congenital heart disease. *Circulation.* 1997;96(9 Suppl):II-346-351.

Ammash N, Warnes C. Cerebrovascular events in adult patients with cyanotic congenital heart disease. *J Am Coll Cardiol*. 1996;28:768-772.

Benza RL, Rayburn BK, Tallaj JA, et al. Efficacy of bosentan in a small cohort of adult patients with pulmonary arterial hypertension related to congenital heart disease. *Chest*. 2006;129:1009-1015.

Fernandes SM, Newburger JW, Lang P, et al. Usefulness of epoprostenol therapy in the severely ill adolescent/adult with Eisenmenger physiology. *Am J Cardiol*. 2003;91:632-635.

Galie N, Beghetti M, Gatzoulis MA, et al. Bosentan therapy in patients with Eisenmenger syndrome: a multicenter, double-blind, randomized, placebo-controlled study. *Circulation*. 2006;114:48-54.

Granton JT, Rabinovitch M. Pulmonary arterial hypertension in congenital heart disease. *Cardiol Clin*. 2002. 20:441-457.

Humpl T, Reyes JT, Holtby H, et al. Beneficial effect of oral sildenafil therapy on childhood pulmonary arterial hypertension: twelve-month clinical trial of a single-drug, open-label, pilot study. *Circulation*. 2005;111:3274-3280.

Oechslin E. Hematological management of the cyanotic adult with congenital heart disease. *Int J Cardiol*. 2004;97(Suppl 1):109-115

Perloff JK, Marelli AJ, Miner PD. Risk of stroke in adults with cyanotic congenital heart disease.[see comment]. *Circulation*. 1993;87:1954-1959.

Rosenzweig EB, Kerstein D, Barst RJ. Long-term prostacyclin for pulmonary hypertension with associated congenital heart defects. *Circulation*. 1999;99:1858-1865.

Schulze-Neick I, Gilbert N, Ewert R, et al. Adult patients with congenital heart disease and pulmonary arterial hypertension: first open prospective multicenter study of bosentan therapy. *Am Heart J*. 2005;150:716.

Singh TP, Rohit M, Grover A, et al. A randomized, placebo-controlled, double-blind, crossover study to evaluate the efficacy of oral sildenafil therapy in severe pulmonary artery hypertension. *Am Heart J*. 2006;151:851.e1-5.

Vongpatanasin W, Brickner ME, Hillis LD, et al. The Eisenmenger syndrome in adults. *Ann Intern Med*,. 1998;128:745-755.

CASE 32: TETRALOGY OF FALLOT—SELECTED REFERENCES

Anderson RH, Weinberg. The clinical anatomy of tetralogy of Fallot. Cardiol Young. 2005 15;38-47. . .

Child JS. "Fallot's tetralogy and pregnancy: prognostication and prophesy". *J. Am. Coll. Cardiol.* **44** (1): 181–3.

Eldadah ZA, Hamosh A, Biery NJ, et al. "Familial Tetralogy of Fallot caused by mutation in the jagged1 gene". *Hum. Mol. Genet.* **10** (2): 163–9.

Gatzoulis MA, Webb GD, Daubeney PE. Diagnosis and Management of Adult Congenital Heart Disease. Churchill Livingstone, Philadelphia. Goldmuntz E, Geiger E, Benson DW. "NKX2.5 mutations in patients with tetralogy of Fallot". *Circulation.* **104** (21): 2565–8

Guntheroth WG, Mortan BC, Mullins GL, Baum D. Am Venous return with knee-chest position and squatting in tetralogy of Fallot. Heart J. 1968 Mar;75(3):313-8.

Lillehei CW; Cohen, M; Warden, HE; Read, RC; Aust, JB; Dewall, RA; Varco, RL . "Direct Vision Intracardiac Surgical Correction of the Tetralogy of Fallot, Pentalogy of Fallot, and Pulmonary Atresia Defects Report of First Ten Cases". *Ann. Surg.* **142** (3): 418–442. .

Murakami T. "Squatting: the hemodynamic change is induced by enhanced aortic wave reflection". *Am. J. Hypertens.* **15** (11): 986–8.

Tsze DS, Vitberg YM, Berezow J, Starc TJ, Dayan PS (2014). "Treatment of tetralogy of fallot hypoxic spell with intranasal fentanyl". *Pediatrics.* **134** (1): e266–9.

Warnes, Carole A. "The Adult With Congenital Heart Disease". *Journal of the American College of Cardiology.* **46** (1): 1–8. .

CASE 40: PULMONARY STENOSIS

Hameed AB, Goodwin TM, Elkayam U. Effect of pulmonary stenosis on pregnancy outcomes--a case-control study. *Am Heart J.* November 2007. 154:852. .

Nishimura RA, Otto CM, Bonow RO, Carabello BA, Erwin JP 3rd, Guyton RA, et al. 2014 AHA/ACC Guideline for the Management of Patients With Valvular Heart Disease: a report of the American College of Cardiology/American Heart Association Task Force on Practice Guidelines. *Circulation.* 2014 Jun 10. 129(23):e521-643.

Rios, J.C., Walsh, B., Ewy, G., Marcus, F., and Massumi, R. A.: Congenital pulmonary artery stenosis. *Am. J. Cardiology* 23:318, 1969.

Shaath G, Mutairi MA, Tamimi O, Alakhfash A, Abolfotouh M, Alhabshan F. Predictors of re-intervention in neonates with critical pulmonary stenosis or pulmonary atresia with intact ventricular septum. *Catheter Cardiovasc Interv.* 2011 Sep 27.

T, Taylor AM. Pulmonary valve interventions. *Expert Rev Cardiovasc Ther.* 2011 Nov. 9(11):1445-57.

Vahanian A, Alfieri O, Andreotti F, Antunes MJ, Barón-Esquivias G, Baumgartner H, et al. Guidelines on the management of valvular heart disease (version 2012). *Eur Heart J.* 2012 Oct. 33(19):2451-96.

Warnes CA, Williams RG, Bashore TM, Child JS, Connolly HM, Dearani JA, et al. ACC/AHA 2008 Guidelines for the Management of Adults with Congenital Heart Disease: a report of the American College of Cardiology/American Heart Association Task Force on Practice Guidelines (writing committee to develop guidelines on the management of adults with congenital heart disease). *Circulation.* 2008 Dec 2. 118(23):e714-833.

Zdradzinski MJ, Qureshi AM, Stewart R, et al. Comparison of long-term postoperative sequelae in patients with tetralogy of Fallot versus isolated pulmonic stenosis. *Am J Cardiol.* 2014 Jul 15. 114(2):300-4

INDEX

A

Acute rheumatic fever (ARF), 19, 28
adenosine, 86
afterload, 4, 12–13, 34, 36, 42, 73, 80, 93, 148
American College of Cardiology (ACC), 25
American Heart Association, 25
aneurysm, 56, 119–20
 ventricular, vi, 116–17, 333
angina pectoris
 stable, 84–85, 87, 91, 93, 98
 unstable, 97, 149
angioplasty, 94
Anticoagulation, 111, 124, 214, 270, 275
aorta, 11, 56, 60, 77, 313
aortic dissection, 56, 76–77, 80
aortic stenosis, 54–56, 59–62, 72, 80
 severe, 60, 64
 valvular, 54–56
aortic valve, 57–58, 62–63, 67–68, 71
 bicuspid, 56
Aortic valve sclerosis (AVS), 56
arrhythmia, 91, 109, 112
 cardiac, 109, 112
 ventricular, 61
atherosclerotic plaque, 89, 99

atrial fibrillation (AF), viii, 23–24, 26, 37, 47, 119, 125, 188, 238, 240, 258, 261, 264–70, 273–77, 354–56
atrioventricular node (AV), 24

B

beta-blockers, 46, 76, 93, 106, 154, 165, 183, 234, 243

C

calcium channel blockers, 93
cardiac catheterization, 36, 39
cardiogenic shock, 41, 139, 337
cardiomyopathy, vii, 43, 55–56, 177, 184, 222, 237, 346, 352
 obstructive, 55–56
catecholamines, 5
compliance, 6, 10–11, 15, 32, 37–38, 40, 52–53, 59–61, 64, 68, 78, 91, 95
 decreased, 6, 10, 60, 91, 95
 increased, 64, 95
contractility, 5–6, 33, 56, 91
coronary angioplasty, 94, 110–11, 141
coronary artery disease, 85–86, 92, 99

coronary disease, 85–86, 98–99, 107
cyanosis, 20

D

diastole, 22–23, 68, 71, 79
diastolic pressure, 10, 87
diastolic rumble, 22, 295
dilatation, 35, 52, 57, 69, 71, 104
dyspnea, 20, 69

E

echocardiogram, 19, 29, 45, 49–50, 92
echocardiography, 3, 9, 23, 35, 62, 72, 346
edema, 18, 20, 24, 27–28, 32, 40, 42, 44, 52, 61, 78
  pulmonary, 18, 20, 24, 27, 40, 61, 78
ejection, 58
ejection fraction (EF), 10, 68
endocarditis, 25, 81

F

Fallot, tetralogy of, 48, 316, 319

G

glycolysis, 100, 102

H

heart failure, 46, 61, 68

  congestive (CHF), 50, 52, 107
hypertension, 23–24, 77, 84
  essential, 76, 85
  pulmonary, ix, 19, 23–24, 41, 52, 290, 296, 302, 304–6, 360
hypertrophy, 1, 18–19, 23–24, 29, 33, 35, 38, 45, 49, 54, 59, 61, 81, 88, 104, 290
  ventricular, 1, 45, 49, 54
hypotension, 41, 87, 145, 157
  orthostatic, vii, 157–59, 340

I

ischemia, 38, 59, 61, 70, 78, 87, 90–92, 100, 102
  subendocardial, 59, 70, 78, 91–92

L

lesions, 60–61, 94

M

mitral stenosis, 18–19
mitral valve, 15, 20–24, 29–30, 45–46, 67, 71, 75
mitral valve prolapse (MVP), 45–46, 67
murmur, 3, 22–23, 28, 35, 38, 42, 46, 48–52, 54, 57, 60, 66, 71, 76–77, 79, 97
  cardiac, 1, 7, 28
  diastolic, 31, 33, 66, 71, 76, 79
  ejection, 7–8, 14, 54, 56, 71–72
  functional, 9

pansystolic, 28, 39
systolic, 1, 3, 31, 45, 50, 54, 66, 76, 291
myocardial contractility, 2, 6, 44, 74
myocardial infarction
  acute, vi, 40, 97–101, 106, 108–9, 144, 332
  acute inferior, 39, 97
  ST elevation, 106, 109, 146
myocardial ischemia, vi, 61, 70, 83, 86–87, 90
myocardium, 86–87, 89–92, 102

P

pacemaker, 4, 234
palpitations, 46, 238, 272, 293
peripheral vascular resistance (PVR), 11
plaque rupture, 99–100, 110–11, 152
preload, 13, 34, 110
presystolic accentuation, 18, 23
prostaglandins, 2
pulmonary vascular resistance (PVR), 2, 11–12, 112, 300

R

regurgitation
  acute aortic, 77–80
  acute mitral, 32, 35, 39–42
  chronic mitral, v, 28–30, 32, 34, 37–38, 40, 42
  mitral, 10, 25, 28–29, 32, 34–36, 40, 45

tricuspid, v, 15, 24, 49–53, 272, 329
reperfusion, 102, 105, 110, 141
right coronary artery (RCA), 87, 101

S

stroke index, 10
stroke volume, 2–4, 7, 9–10, 21, 33, 40–41, 43–44, 53, 57, 60–61, 64–65, 68, 71, 78, 103, 117
syndrome
  acute coronary (ACS), 99
  Marfan, 66–67, 78
systole, 4, 6, 9–10, 30, 34–35, 38–39, 42, 45–46, 55, 57, 60, 88

T

Tachycardia, 88, 201, 204, 213, 352
tachycardia, ventricular (VT), 352
therapy, thrombolytic, 107, 111
transaortic percutaneous replacement, 73
turbulence, 8–9, 57–58, 61, 71, 205

V

Valsalva, 46
vasoconstriction, 11–12, 23, 35, 41, 44, 88, 122–23, 138, 152, 181
vasodilation, 11–13

www.ingramcontent.com/pod-product-compliance
Lightning Source LLC
Chambersburg PA
CBHW020625220526
45464CB00001B/23